THE BEAUTY GIRLS

A Floundering Woman's Midlife Career Change to Beauty School

Carol Leonard
Bad Beaver Publishing
Hopkinton, NH

Photos on pages 73, 109, 143 courtesy of Esthetics Institute, Inc., Concord, NH. Cover photo of Kudra MacCaillech and all other photos are property of Bad Beaver Publishing, 2009. All line drawings by Carol Leonard.

Bad Beaver Publishing
585 Hopkinton Road
Hopkinton, NH 03229
603.224.4596
www.badbeaverpublishing.com

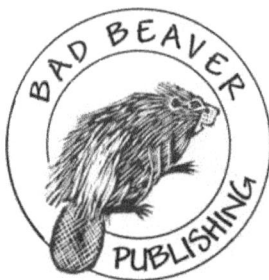

Library of Congress Cataloging-in-Publication Data
Leonard, Carol
The beauty girls/ Carol Leonard.
p.cm
ISBN 978-0-615-33602-2

Second Printing [with 18 Illustrations]

Also by Carol Leonard

Lady's Hands, Lion's Heart, A Midwife's Saga

The Circle of Life
(Co-authored with Elizabeth Davis)

Women of the Thirteenth Moon,
A Baby Boomer's Survival Guide to Menopause

Medea

The Making of Bad Beaver Farm

Dedications

~)(~

This book is dedicated to my little sister, Wendy Leonard Hayes, who suffered through my Beauty School debacle as my "test rat". She stoically volunteered to be my "practice model" for my licensing exam and sat patiently while I did her make-up. Unfortunately, the end result looked frighteningly like Joan Crawford. Wendy is also the genius who came up with the fabulous name "Wraps & Paps." Thank you, Sistah. You are the original Beauty Girl!

And…I want to thank my dear husband, Tom Lajoie, for his saint-like patience with my severe postmenopausal insomnia while writing this book. I so appreciate him for not kicking me out of bed when I was laughing like a hyena and getting up to write while remembering the previous day's events.

I love you Tom…you are a precious rock.

Table of Contents

Prologue:

The Hot Flash Row

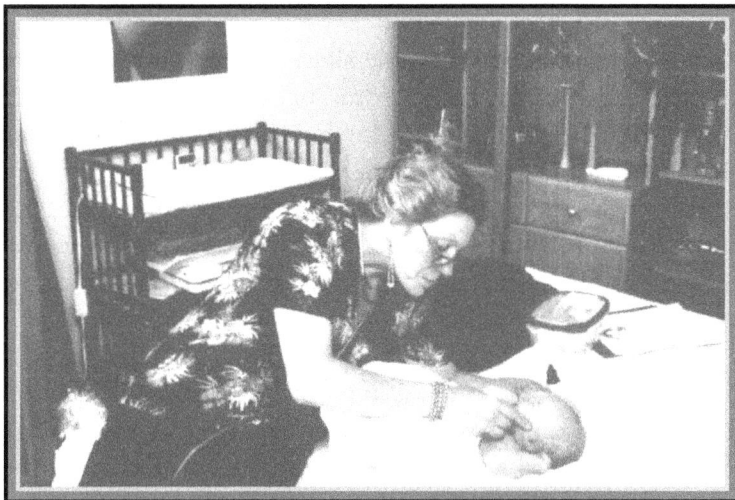

~)(~

PROLOGUE

Winter 2005 ~ I close my thriving birth center due to lack of third party reimbursement and it damn near breaks my heart. It is a beautiful facility that has a fabulous reputation and I can't make a go of it without insurance coverage. It makes no sense for the insurance companies to refuse to cover us...we save them a ton of money, but they refuse anyway and drive us out of business.

The bastards.

I retire from catching babies and wander around aimlessly. I have been a midwife for thirty years and I love my profession more than life itself. I was the first midwife in New

Hampshire and have delivered a bazillion kids but I don't really have any other employable skills. I garden and take care of our farm. I spend the day in my brown velour sweats and crack my first beer of the day for lunch and email legislators about shitty legislation to make myself feel productive.

I know my husband Tom is concerned about me, but he never says much more than, "Honey, I've always loved you in brown." What a great guy. He's a survivor. He knows how to protect himself from great bodily harm.

I start to get worried about me too. The physical hygiene has been definitely slipping. I garden all day, am coated with dirt and sweat. I fall asleep for the night dirty without bothering to shower. When I look in the mirror in the morning, I see a wild postmenopausal woman with edematous, fluid-filled sacs under her eyes looking back.

My scrotum eyes.

I have been able to get by for fifty-five years on a great smile, good genes and a diet of nutritious food and lots of wine…but now I am starting to seriously look like the functional bag lady I really am; no question. This is bad, something's got to give, but I have no idea what.

~)(~

Late Summer 2005 ~ I am sitting in my car on Main Street, Concord, pissed that I have yet another parking ticket. Soon I'm going to get the proverbial Boot. Concord has the worst frustrating parking problem. I look up to see a marquee that says:

ESTHETICS INSTITUTE FOR
ADVANCED SKIN CARE
~ Enroll now for Fall Classes starting in September ~

I sit there looking at the sign until I wonder if I've had a stroke. Can't move. Yeah, right. You're contemplating going to Beauty School. You are desperate, girl. Wicked desperate.

Yeah? Well, listen, Scrotum Eyes…how's this sound? The thing you loved the most about the Birth Center was the "Spa" aspect…the sense of community, the sense of a beautiful place where women could go for their health care and feel included and be heard and respected…not a cold medical/clinical environment to be dreaded but a delicious place to be pampered and take care of one's necessary Whole Woman health regimen.

Epiphany 101 ~ I start to grin as the concept begins to develop. Right! I could get licensed as an Esthetician and open a Spa. Women can come in for their annual exams…and have a yummy facial and get checked under the hood. They can have breast exams, seaweed algae wraps, lash tinting, blood work, Pap smears! Brazilians! The Works! After a woman has her pelvic exam and her feet are in stirrups…she can have a pedicure! I am on fire. I will name my Spa…

WRAPS & PAPS!

OK…I'm gonna do it. I'm going to Beauty School.

I tell Tom that I plan to enroll in Beauty School. I can feel his eyes bore right through me. I know he thinks I won't last one week. But being the gentleman he is, he doesn't say this.

Instead he says, "Do whatever you want to do…because I know you will anyway." I know the boy has serious reservations.

I tell my friends I'm thinking about going to Beauty School. They say, "You've got to be kidding." I say, No, listen, I want to open a Holistic Health Spa for Natural Women's Healthcare. They make fun of me. They say I'm

15

going to be surrounded by vacuous nineteen year olds. I don't care; I think the idea is genius.

I go to the school to check it out. It is a huge old green Victorian house that has been converted to a clinic in the front and classrooms in the back. The main classroom is two stories high and looks like a basketball court. It has a walkway around the second floor that looks like it's for the Wardens. There are a few women in white lab coats huddled around a table in the back eating chocolate. They look bored out of their minds.

I am given a "Complimentary Facial" for prospective students. An Instructor supervises the service. The Instructor is a full-figured blond with short spiky hair and twinkling blue eyes. She's probably a little younger than I. She reminds me of my sister. The student's touch is timid and starts to get annoying but I don't say anything. The Instructor gently corrects her a couple of times. She tells the student I have "mature" skin. I think that's a very diplomatic way of saying I'm aging quickly. Well, at least something about me is mature.

The Instructor asks if I am a midwife. I say Yes, how did she know? She says by my email address--"CLmidwife."

She asks why I want to come to school and I say because I can't tolerate being on-call anymore. It's funny because this is the first time I have admitted that. She says she knows the feeling because she used to be a respiratory therapist and couldn't stand the night call anymore either. I like her immediately.

I meet with the owner. The owner looks a little like Nancy Reagan. She has had so many facelifts she looks like a dog sticking its head out of the window of a car going sixty. The owner knows me. I ask her if I would be the oldest woman ever to enroll and she laughs. She tells me lots of women have "mid-life career changes." I think, "You mean mid-life crisis." She is pleasant and sweet and encouraging. I take a deep breath, make the financial arrangements and sign up for 600 hours.

~)(~

September 2005 ~ It is the night before the first day of school. I toss and turn and can't sleep. I'm nervous as hell. What the hell am I doing anyway? What am I out of my mind? I have never put anything on my face except Ivory Soap and Nivea. Beauty School? Yeeesh.

Around 3:00 in the morning I realize I forgot to make my lunch. I get up, take one of Tom's insulated beer coolers with a contractor's logo on it and make a snack. I pack leftover salmon and rice and tomatoes from the garden. Little School Girl.

When I finally do fall asleep, I have an anxiety dream that I have overslept and have missed the first day of school. I realize it has been approximately forty years since I last had that dream.

When I am getting dressed for school, Tom sings "Beauty School Drop-Out" to me at the top of his lungs. I have to wear a "uniform" of black shoes, black pants and a white top. I have been instructed to wear "subtle" make-up. Jesus.

I walk in the front door of the clinic side of the school. There are two other women nervously waiting. They are both wearing the requisite black and white student outfit. One woman is of indeterminate age; the other is around my age. Definitely around my age, if not older. She is non-descript and pudgy. They seem friendly. I relax a little bit.

It is 8:30 AM. More women start pouring in. They are pretty silent. Some are whispering. We are herded up to the

"Trainee" classroom in the back where we will be sequestered for the next eight weeks. My class is huge—two times the normal size. There are twelve of us. I am in the middle row with the Woman of Indeterminate Age and the Pudgy One sitting to my left. The seats are filling up. At the last minute a buxom brunette with spiky hair and purple eye shadow rushes in and sits to my right. She's around my age too.

The women in the row in front of us are all in their early twenties and are all drop-dead gorgeous. I mean seriously gorgeous in a healthy, glowing, long blond hair, classic Christie Brinkley kind of way. I turn around. The women in the row in back of us are also all in their early twenties with the same stunningly attractive, classy "Town & Country" kind of blond, blinding white teeth, All-American natural beauty.

All except for the young dark haired woman at the end of the row with the eyebrows shaved off. Her hair is short and teased and her eyebrows are penciled in high and arched. She reminds me of Divine in "Pink Flamingo." She has a black tattoo on her neck. She shoots me a dark look like, "What the hell are you looking at?" I whip back around in my seat. She scares the shit out of me.

I begin to get incredibly hot. I ask the women in my row if it's really hot in here or is it just me? The Woman of Indeterminate Age says, "No, you're having a hot flash." She laughs and says, "Me too."

The instructor comes in. It is the same zaftig woman I met before. I am happy to see her. Her name is Sophie and we are going to be stuck with her for the first eight weeks of our curriculum. We go around the room doing introductions. Most of the women are in the "food service industry," are waitresses and want to get out of "dead end jobs."

The Pudgy woman next to me is a Zen Buddhist and the Brunette is a Nail Tech. The Dark Haired One in the back row is a bartender and says her goal is to make tons of money doing make-up for the strippers before they do their routines in the Combat Zone in Boston. I turn around and grin at her. This girl has balls. Her name is Vivienne.

Our Instructor, Sophie, is telling us the rules. We must be here and signed in promptly at 8:30 AM or the door will be closed and we will be locked out until lunchtime. We will be signed out at 4:30 PM. No chewing gum, hair will be pulled back neatly away from our faces, no dangling jewelry, subtle makeup must be worn at all times. Plain black, soft-soled shoes only, no heels. Lab coats must be pressed, no wrinkles allowed—ever. She asks that we not change our seats so she can remember our names. Some of the young women are taking notes.

In the middle of all this I get poked in the side. It's the buxom brunette with the purple eye shadow.

She says, "You have my pen."

I look down. Damn, I do. I hand it to her, "Sorry."

She rolls her eyes and does a big dramatic sigh. She levels me with a bold, confrontational stare. I can hear her thinking, "Shit. This is gonna be a looong six months."

At the last minute before the door slams shut, a very young, very tiny, dark haired kid sneaks in the back and quietly slides in to the last empty seat. I grin to myself. We're all here. I'm exactly where I'm supposed to be.

I am in the Hot Flash Row.

Week One:

In the Convent Again

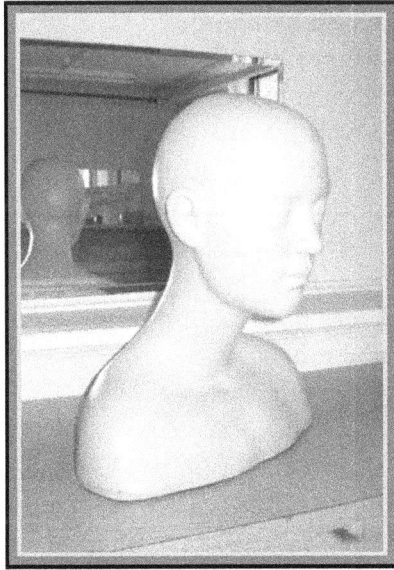

Meet Veronica:
Vivienne's Mannequin

~)(~

Chapter 1

Every morning at 8:31 at the Esthetics Institute we have "Assembly." All the students gather in the big fluorescent-lit two-story room to listen to the Director of Clinical Studies and the Instructors tell us the day's agenda.

The Seniors are with us for this part, then they go out front to work in the clinic. The Director is standing in front of the Head Table welcoming us, the new September class, to the school. She has flawless skin, is probably in her early sixties, and while I can see her lips smiling, her eyes do not. The Director has steel behind those eyes.

I am starting to get that nagging, disorienting feeling that accompanies de'ja vu. I have been here before. I know this scene all too well. Then I remember. In the late Sixties I attended a Catholic girls' college.

How I got there in the Convent, not being a Catholic, is another story. Suffice it to say, however, I got kicked out after three months for insubordination, disobeying all the rules, smoking dope, not wearing a bra, etc. The Director is reminding me of the Mother Superior. I am in the Convent again. This does not bode well.

I make it to Friday. I have not dropped out yet despite Tom's singing "Beauty School Drop-Out" to me every single morning. I am unbelievably excited that it's the weekend and I am going to be out of this room. One week down and only nineteen more to go. Moving right along.

We are sitting in our seats listening to Sophie instruct us as to the proper techniques for Cleansing, Toning and Moisturizing the skin. We are going to work on each other for the first time this afternoon. I am starting to space out. I get poked in the side again; it's my neighbor, Bette, the big brunette with the purple eye shadow and the gorgeous earrings.

She points to my hand. She's angry. She says, "You have my pen."

I look down. Damn, I do. Again. I hand it to her, "Shit. Sorry."

She rolls her eyes and does a big dramatic sigh. She growls, "What the fuck?"

Yow! I turn away but out of the corner of my eye I see Bette crack a smile. Then she cracks a huge smile and laughs out loud.

"Really had you going didn't I?" she says.

24

"Dammit, Bette, you scared the crap out of me."

She's laughing a huge, wide open-mouth laugh now. I realize she has a beautiful smile, her whole face lights up. She's absolutely cracking her own self up. She really is lovely, sort of a cross between Ricki Lake and the young Elizabeth Taylor. I give her another damn pen. She is still laughing.

It's afternoon and we are preparing to Cleanse, Tone and Moisturize each other. Bette and I pair up. One of us is absent today, so Vivienne has to work on a mannequin. The mannequin is only rubber shoulders, neck and bald head. It is left over from when the school was a cosmetology school and they used to do hair. Vivienne names her mannequin Veronica.

The Trainee room is lined with bare facial beds called tables. Sophie has instructed us as to how to properly drape and prepare our tables and heat and fold our towels. Of the paired students, one of us is to be the Client and one the Esthetician. We are to do this professionally and prepare our products to use on each other as though this were the real thing. We are instructed to begin.

Bedlam ensues. Towels are flying everywhere. Hand sanitizer squirts across the room. Someone laughs and calls that the "Money Shot."

I hear a "What the *fuckin' shit*? You dumb ho *bitch*!" from the next table. Nikita.

Nikita is a beautiful blue-eyed blond with long thick curly streaked hair. She has freckles and a cute nose, looks like an innocent Barbie until she opens her mouth. Nikita has the mouth of a trucker.

I'm standing in the middle of a holocaust...my class is so noisy we can barely hear Sophie who is yelling, "Ladies! LADIES! Please!" Finally she yells, "SHUT...UUUP!" The din settles down to a dull roar.

Sophie looks over the top of her glasses and mutters to herself, "Holy Mother of God."

Vivienne raises her hand.

Sophie nods to her, "Yes, Vivienne?"

"My client, Veronica, has issues." She puts a protective hand on her mannequin's shoulder. "She's very sensitive about her height. You know, being so vertically challenged and all. She's feeling like she's being laughed at all the time. Also, between you and me...I'm beginning to think she may be anorexic."

The whole class explodes all over again. Sophie gives up, tells us we're done for the day. I am so happy to get out of there for the weekend. It's weird, but as I sign out and realize I'll be away for three whole days...I kind of feel like I'll miss these guys.

Week Two:

Gorbachev's Forehead

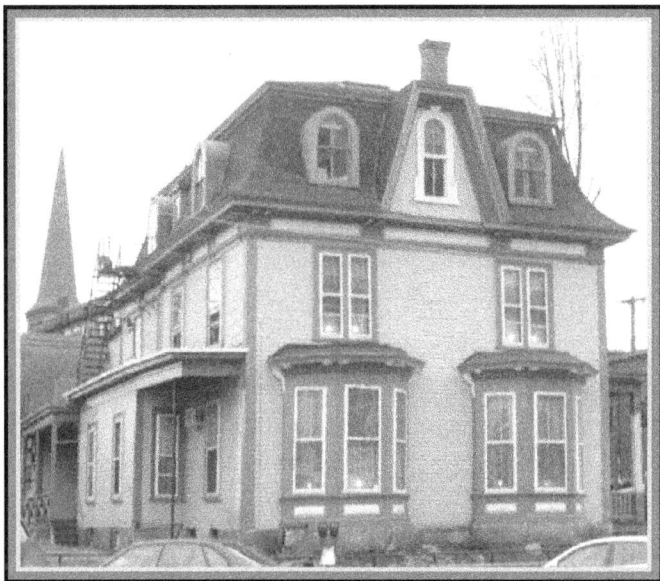

The Convent

~)(~

Chapter 2

Back in the Convent for Round Two. It's starting to fall into a predictable routine. Tests every morning on our assigned Chapter, followed by a lecture with practical hands-on treatments in the afternoon.

On Tuesday we exfoliate. I have never exfoliated in my life, and it probably shows. Fifty-five years of built up sludge. Yick. Some of my classmates exfoliate every day—which seems a little excessive since their skin is so young and dewy; I can't imagine they have any excess smegma to get rid of.

We also learn Skin Analysis under the "Loupe" which is an intense magnifying lamp that magnifies the face to help estheticians analyze and treat the skin. I'm analyzing Nikita's face with this light and the first time I see this big honking zit on her chin, I almost scream. Under the Loupe, the zit looks like a veritable volcano. Terrifying.

~)(~

On Wednesday, after the test on the Physiology and Histology of the Skin, which several of my Peeps tanked, they are in rare form at lunch. They are blowing off tension from the morning.

Nikita is holding court, describing her typical morning before leaving for school. The stream of obscenities is like a tsunami. She imitates her boyfriend, Wes, getting up in the morning. She stands up and scratches her package, then raises her arm to sniff her armpit. She "fake" burps, farts, then says in a low voice,

"Hey, morning Babe."

Then she says, "I'm taking a shower in the downstairs bathroom. There are two bathrooms in our house, but that motherfucker has to come in to where I am to drop the kids off at the pool. Stinks up the whole place 'til I gag."

I have never heard that particular expression. It may be fifth grade bathroom humor but I am laughing so hard I have tears streaming down my face. Our whole class is laughing so hard the sound is deafening.

Nikita imitates her boyfriend sending her off to school. She scratches her crotch again, says he scratches his bubblegum, then fake farts, says, "See ya, Babe. Love you." Burp.

30

I laugh so hard I feel like I am going to throw up. The Beauty Girls are screaming now, big huge open mouths full of food and tonsils. For one brief moment, the September class has become a collective, synchronized alien entity. Our sounds reverberate in the big cavernous gymnasium of a room until it is overwhelming.

I look over to the Head Table. The instructors are looking at us with their mouths dropped open. Mother Superior scowls. They look worried. The September class is out-of-control.

~)(~

On Thursday we learn massage. We are licensed to massage only from the shoulders up. The massage routine we learn is one the Institute has standardized and it's nice. I learned massage from the yoga center, Kripalu, two decades ago and this is very similar. I feel comfortable with this and it is healing and gentle and rhythmic. I feel I am good at it.

On Friday we do our first mask. The mask is "Moor Mud," supposedly from the moors of Transylvania or somewhere and theoretically has great restorative powers. It is dark and thick and I get the shit everywhere. I call it Petrified Donkey Dung and am not real sure I want it on my face. This will take some practice.

It is Friday afternoon. 60 hours down—540 to go. But who's counting?

On the weekend, I experiment by making my own beauty "products" at home, even though we are warned to never do this. I, of course, am defiant and start mixing up all kinds of toners and masks in my kitchen. I am having a ball putting various concoctions on my face. My own all-natural line of beauty products. My favorite invention is:

Cleansing Kitchen Mask
2 Green Tea Bags
½ C Oats
1 t Baking Soda
1 T Honey
½ Avocado, mashed
1 egg
1 T Plain Yogurt

Open the tea bags and let steep in a little warm water to cover. Combine everything else together and pour in enough Green Tea to make a mush. Apply immediately to clean skin and leave on for 10 to 15 minutes. Rinse off with warm water. Do not lie down with this mask on anyplace where there may be ants.

The milk from the oats contains salicylic acid to soothe the skin, and the baking soda leaves your skin silky smooth. The Cleansing Kitchen Mask gives the skin a good dose of vitamins, proteins, antioxidants, lecithin and essential fatty acids. You can eat the rest.

That weekend, I get the fabulous idea to try putting pomegranate on my face. Fruit acids are all the "industry buzz," and pomegranate in particular. I grind up fresh pomegranate seeds in my food processor. I apply to my face and leave on for 15 minutes. I rinse. It does not come off. My face is stained a rich Port Wine color that will not wash off. My entire face looks like Mikhail Gorbachev's forehead. It lasts for twenty-four hours. I decide to leave the chemistry to the pros.

Week Three:

Shrimpy's Hysterectomy

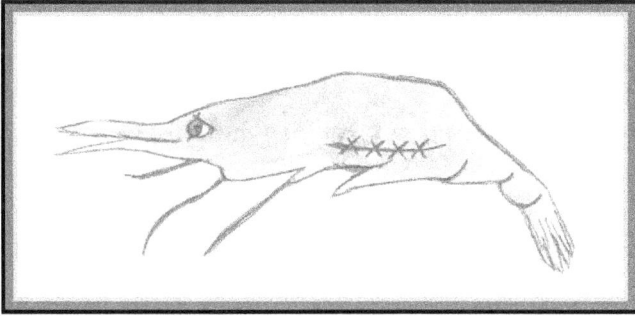

Shrimpy's Hysterectomy

~)(~

Chapter 3

The little dark-haired kid has taken to following me around. I'm not sure why exactly, but every time I turn around, there she is. Her name is Crystal but I call her Shrimpy because she weighs ninety pounds soaking wet.

Shrimpy and I are walking down the block to the local pizza place to grab something for lunch. It's nice to be outside, away from the fluorescent lights.

She looks up at me and says, "I want to ask you a question."

I say, "OK shoot."

"Do you smoke dope?" she asks.

Ah, so that's it, she has figured out that I am an Old Hippie.

I think back to the last times I smoked, and the anxiety attacks and how paranoid I got and how extremely unpleasant that all was.

"Nope. I haven't smoked in thirty-five years."

"Thirty-five years! That's how old my mother is!"

I stop in my tracks. That means her mother was born after the whole protesting the Vietnam War era. Her mother. I don't know what to say.

I say, "Shrimpy, I lived a whole lifetime before your mother was even born."

This week we are studying Diseases and Disorders of the Skin. It's pretty interesting. We are also learning about electricity and "machines" that are used in skin care, and I hate it. I just can't get with the whole machine thing. It all sounds so preposterous. Anaphoresis and iotophoresis and Galvanic current. And saponification—this is a chemical reaction that "transforms" the sebum of the skin into soap...soap! This sounds like utter bullshit to me. Hocus-pocus. I realize I don't give a rat's ass about any of it. I flunk the test.

Shrimpy is reading a book about hysterectomy. I sit down and ask, what's up with that?

She says after she's done having kids, she's going to do it. Have a hysterectomy.

I'm trying hard not to laugh. "Oh, really? Why is that?"

She says the pain with her periods is unbearable. She's seen a bunch of doctors about it but nothing helps. I say let's talk about your diet for a minute.

"What'd you eat yesterday?"

"Some crackers, an orange, two things of Ramen noodles. And a glass of milk."

"Well, the milk is good. That's a start. How about anything for protein?"

We talk about easy ways for her to get more protein in her diet. Cheese, beans, tuna fish. She says she'll write down everything she eats for a week for me to look at. I tell her that increasing the amount of protein she gets daily might improve a lot of stuff with her. She promises to pay more attention and try harder to eat better. Hysterectomy. Yeesh.

On Wednesday I have to leave school early to testify at a legislative hearing for the Midwives Bill to mandate insurance coverage for freestanding birth centers. I've been fighting this battle since I had to close my facility last winter. When I get to the State House I learn that the insurance lobbyists have lied…again! Our bill is to be tabled for "study." I am so angry, I swear I burst a blood vessel in my head. I get a killer migraine that makes me vomit every time I move my head. I am sick all night. I miss school the next day.

I am lying in bed in the late afternoon and I am feeling a little better. I am thinking about school. I am thinking about dropping out. Some of it seems so vacuous. It just doesn't have the rush that midwifery has…doesn't have the thrill, the drama, the intensity. I'm thinking maybe I've made a huge mistake.

My phone rings. It's Bette. She's calling from school to see how I'm doing.

"That's sweet of you Bette, it's really nice to hear your voice."

I hear this god-awful sound in the background. It sounds like a barnyard.

"What the hell is that noise?"

She holds out her phone. It's deafening.

"It's them. The girls."

"Oh my god. That's frightening."

"Yeah, well, par for the course. For some reason the energy level in here is really high this afternoon. They're all getting ready to leave."

I can just picture Vivienne doing her little Curly from the Three Stooges backward hopping. She's really good at it. She says she practices.

I grin. I listen some more. I know that sound. It sounds like birds. Hundreds of migrating grackles landing in a tree, squawking.

"That's awesome."

Bette says, "What? What's that? Can't hear you. Gotta go. Bye."

I laugh. The Beauty Girls. Excited to be out of there. Most of them will go to their waitressing jobs and will work until midnight. Then they'll go home and study and then get up for the 8:30 class and do it all over again. Some of them have to drive a fair distance. I don't know how they do it. Getting by on a few hours sleep.

Yes I do.

They're young.

~)(~

The next day I do end up going back to school...but Bette is out. All that the Instructors say is that she had an accident. I panic, thinking she may have had a car crash or something so I call her from our lunch tables on my cell.

She answers with a muffled "hello." She's lying on her couch with an ice pack on her head. It turns out that she was throwing a Kong for her big German Shepherd and as she was reaching down to pick it up, her running dog barreled straight into her and they cracked heads. He knocked her out for a second.

I laugh. "You mean to say your dog knocked you out?"

"Yep. Out cold."

One of the Beauty Girls, Pearl, overhears this conversation. She makes an announcement to the whole class;

"Bette's dog knocked her up."

Dead silence. Everyone is staring at her in disbelief.

She says it again, emphatically. "Bette's dog knocked her up."

I yell at her, "Pearl, Pearl, I said OUT not UP!"

"Oh."

I tell Bette what Pearl just said.

Bette sighs and says, "She's number than a pounded thumb, that girl."

We hang up.

Knocked up…for *chrissake*.

~)(~

On the last day of the week we learn to do extractions, which is a more scientific sounding term for popping everyone's zits. The Beauty Girls are way into this. I haven't had a pimple in about forty years so I'm left extractionless. They go at it with a vengeance. Someone says they find it a little nauseating. I'm thinking to myself it's a toss-up for me as a midwife, between this and treating yeast infections or BV.

I spare the Beauty Girls the drippy details.

Another week down…*seventeen* to go. Time flies when you're having fun.

Week Four:
The Panty Party

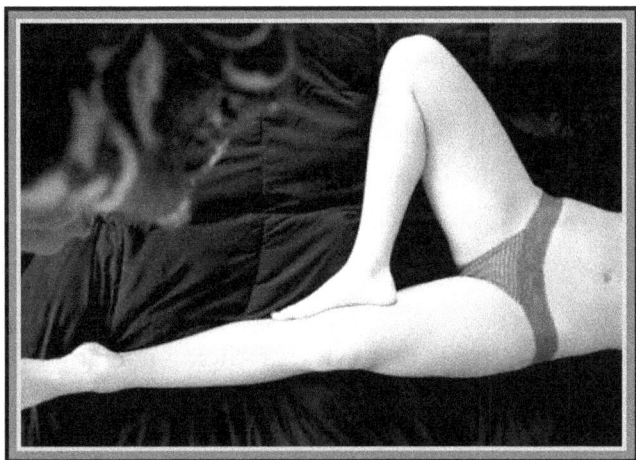

The Figure 4 Position

~)(~

Chapter 4

Sugaring.

The whole week is devoted to learning the art of Body Sugaring. It's actually pretty cool and I grow to like it. It is an Ancient Art of hair removal and it works with just sugar and water and lemon juice. Hard to believe, but that rips the hair right out and doesn't tear the skin. Supposedly, it's much gentler on the skin than hard wax and it absolutely is easier to work with.

Sophie instructs us how to prepare the skin for the sugaring with cleansing, drying and powdering. Then she demonstrates how to coat a thin film of warm sugar, which has the consistency and appearance of honey, on with our spatulas in the direction of hair growth. Then we take some Pellon fabric strips and place over the area to be sugared and rub it quickly to warm it up, again in the direction of the hair. Then we >>>*Schwip!*>>>rip the strip at a 45 degree angle against the grain of the hair—and it all comes out. Smooth as a baby's bottom.

The Beauty Girls are all over this like ants on honey. They can't wait to be sugared. They've been storing up all their hair just for this day. They were instructed to *not shave* since day one of school and they all believe they are hairy beasts. They are showing their legs and their pits in some kind of estrogen driven competition to see who is the most hirsute. They have not bared their legs or their underarms to their boyfriends in over three weeks.

I can't see anyone's hair. All I see is adorable light little downy peach fuzz. Bette and I walk down to CVS and I get a new pair of glasses. I bump up the magnification a couple of levels to 1.75 and I find some fabulous purple glasses that I love. When I come back to the Sugar Shack, I can see a few more hairs but mostly I think they all have pathological aversions to body hair.

Except for Nikita. She really is hairy, yikes. She is walking around with her fuzzy legs exposed making Wookie sounds like Chewbacca. WRAAHWW! She does a great imitation. All day for the next week, all I hear is *Schwip! Schwip! Schwip!* as all the hair disappears.

We start with the legs. I don't really have any hair on my legs, never have. I'm sort of like a hairless Chihuahua. But Mary fakes sugaring my legs anyway and it makes them incredibly soft. Her legs are better, much more fun. I can see a ton of hair on the strips after I have *Schwipped* her.

Next to go are the armpits, genteelly referred to as *"Underarms"* at the Institute. I look over at Nikita where they are gathered around her doing her pits. She is in a cold sweat from the pain. They've given up on the regular sugar, tried the next-step-up sugar for "stubborn" hair, and now they're on to the high-test Spa Paste for impossible hair. Nikita looks like she's going to pass out. Her pits look like raw hamburger. I think they may need a crowbar.

I'm doing Mary's underarms, and I say I think it is so ironic to be doing this since I didn't even shave my pits until I was probably in my early forties. I say I was a Hippie Chick and I was proud of my fuzzy underarms; it was some kind of rebellious statement. She says "Me too!" Mary is my seatmate to the left of me in the Hot Flash Row. She is quiet, thoughtful, and smart as hell. She says she lived in a teepee in Colorado for years in the Sixties.

On the day we are to sugar our "bikini lines," all the Beauty Girls have worn their best party panties. I can't believe the scene around me. All the girls are reclined on their tables with their legs splayed open in the "Figure 4" position with the most unbelievable array of festive panties ever imagined. Most are wearing thongs, striped ones, pink ones, one with a big purple sequin butterfly on the front, satin ones, lace ones. All have perfect slender bodies. It looks like some demented porn filmmaker's ultimate fantasy version of "Catholic School Girls Gone Bad."

I'm thinking if Tom were here right now, he'd think he died and gone to Heaven.

I am working with Pearl on this day. I have worn my own favorite party panties…my saucy red velvet thong with the black trim and the black brocade rose on the back. But I'm looking around at everyone else and thinking I am definitely going to have to upgrade my lingerie selection if I'm going to keep up with these wenches.

Pearl has got me beat. She is wearing a black leather thong with beautiful rhinestones along the top edges. She has a fabulous tiny little body. She's a funny kid. The skin on her face is so perfectly translucent and pearly; she looks like a porcelain doll. She has enormous eyes with long dark lashes and the ditziest laugh I have ever heard. She is, quite possibly, the most vacuous person I have ever met. She shows me her tattoos. She has two, one on each hipbone. She explains that they are her birth signs, because she was born exactly on the cusp; she has two Zodiac signs. Pearl is very proud of her tattoos.

Now that we are all finally hairless, some of the girls even sugared their forearms; we are presentable enough to start dealing with the real public. Friday afternoon has been designated "Friends and Family Day" and we will be performing Express Facials on Real People. My mother is my first client; she hasn't left for Florida yet. I'm surprised that I'm actually a little nervous, performance anxiety I guess. I wait at the front door and see my mom coming down the sidewalk. She looks so little to me now. I greet her, help her into her wrap and she hops up on the table.

I analyze my mom's skin—beyond "mature". She has the same telangiectasia that I do from sun damage. I realize I'm probably looking through the loupe at my own skin in twenty-five years. During the massage portion I'm looking at my mom and I am flooded with a totally unexpected wave of tenderness and love for my mother. She is such a great role model. What a great facial—for me. I'm loving this.

I realize with great clarity—I'm having fun now. I'm having one hell of a good time.

Week Five:

The Masturbator Muscle

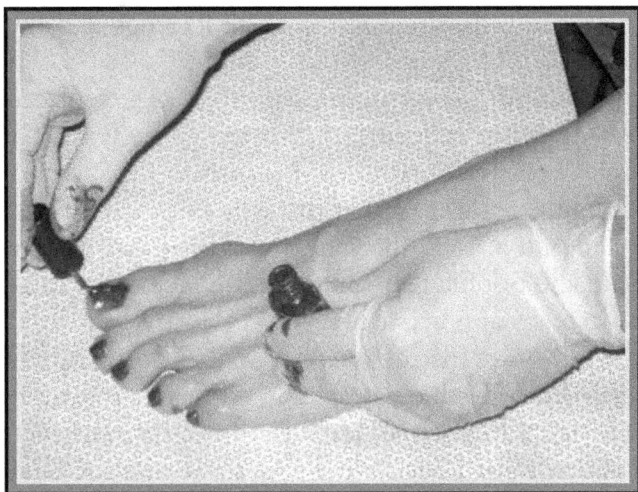

Voted Best Finger Painter in School

~)(~

Chapter 5

I have been in the Convent for over a month. Tom says he's surprised I've stuck it out this long. He says he could tell I was struggling with the decision to stay or leave the day I stayed home from school. He knew it was hard for me to go back. He says he's proud of me. He has stopped singing Beauty School Drop-Out to me.

At the beginning of the week, in Assembly, the Mother Superior tells us that it is officially Fall. After this week we are no longer allowed to wear open-toed shoes. This is akin to the "No White Shoes After Labor Day" rule, I guess. I have been wearing a straight black skirt and tights and open-toed black shoes. My legs are so skinny that the Beauty

Girls tease me about the two Tampon Strings hanging down from my skirt. I find my old favorite black cowboy boots; I dust them off and start wearing black leggings and my black cowboy boots.

We find out that Sophie has been replaced with another Instructor named Jett. We are upset at first because we think she's been replaced because we are so bad and unruly. Sophie assures us that this is the normal schedule. We buy a card and a bottle of wine and a huge bar of extra dark chocolate and Sophie tears up when we give them to her. She knows we really appreciate her.

Our new Instructor Jett is the polar opposite of Sophie. Where Sophie's teaching style was nurturing and encouraging and maternal, Jett's is not. Jett is taut and tightly coiled and commanding. She is like some kind of feral feline about to pounce. She seems to have a lot of suppressed energy ready to be unleashed. Even though she is physically tiny, she carries a big stick. She is ten years younger than I am and does not have one wrinkle anywhere. *None.* She is very disciplined (which is my nice way of saying…she is tightly wrapped.)

Sophie and Jett are best friends; they went to school together at the Convent a long time ago. They are absolute physical contrasts. Sophie is large and blond and soft and approachable, Jett is tiny and dark and firm and authoritative. She has spiky dark hair and chic black glasses. She is actually quite beautiful. I can tell Sophie and Jett really love each other.

I have the feeling Jett is going to expect us to be disciplined too. We may be in big trouble.

This week we are studying Anatomy and Physiology and the Beauty Girls are freaking out. Cells, Tissues, Organs, Body Systems, The Skeletal System, The Muscular System, The Nervous System, The Circulatory System, The Endocrine

System, The Digestive System, The Excretory System, The Respiratory System, The Integumentary System and a little tiny bit of my specialty, The Reproductive System. Jett is ripping right through all of this.

Even though it was a couple of millennia ago, I was a biology major in college, so most of this stuff starts creeping out of the musty, 1960s cobwebs in my brain. I dust off some of the old Latin derivatives and remember some of the root words to the names. I try to show some of my classmates how to figure this out by recognizing certain root words. The Beauty Girls have made flashcards and are constantly quizzing each other in order to memorize muscles, nerves, bones.

Jett is desperately trying to help us get the A&P down rote. She is randomly throwing out terms to quiz us.

"OK, someone. What's the *Sternocleidomastoideus*?"

Nikita says, "That's the muscle in the neck that rotates the head. I love that word… *Sternocleidomastoideus*. That just homeslices."

I say, "You only like it because it has 'STERNO' in it, Nikita."

Jett continues, "OK, what is the Masseter?"

Pearl raises her hand.

Jett says, "Yes, Pearl."

Pearl states, "That's the Masturbator Muscle." Pearl flutters her impossibly long eyelashes.

Jett winces and cocks up one eyebrow. Everyone stares at Pearl dumbfounded.

I realize that we are definitely looking at the shallow end of the gene pool. A little later on, in our lecture on the Nervous System, Pearl interrupts Jett.

Pearl is excited. She says, "OK, like, I think I'm getting this. So, like, the muscles are attached to the bones. And the brain sends a signal down along the nerves to the muscles, and like, then my hand moves. Every time I move, like, this has happened?"

Jett looks stunned for a moment but she recovers quickly.

"Yes, Pearl. Something like that. Very good."

Pearl beams and does her little hiccupy laugh. "Cool. That's sooo totally cool." Pearl has had an epiphany.

Shrimpy has taken my advice and has started eating. And eating. And eating. She has become an eating machine. At lunchtime she mooches food from everyone. She's says, "Ooooh, that looks good, mind if I have a bite?" or "You done with those chips?" or "You gonna eat that crust?" I'm beginning to wonder if she has enough money for food. I go across the street to the bakery and buy a loaf of fresh whole grain bread and go next door to the Co-op for cheese. Shrimpy eats most of it in one sitting.

Under Jett's iron will, we have all knuckled down and are seriously studying our A&P. I am sitting in my seat trying to focus on the material, but I am fidgety and beginning to get cranky. Sometimes I am positive I have ADD. I cannot find my pen. I ask Bette if she has my pen.

She doesn't even look up and growls, "Jesus Christ, no."

What the hell? I look over to my left at Mary, and she has my pen. Quiet Mary who has been witness to all of Bette's and my ongoing squabbles about our stuff. I point to my pen and then I smack her upside the back of her head. She screams and Jett whips around, glaring. I point to Mary.

This week we learn to do pedicures and I absolutely suck at it. The first pedicure I, personally, ever had was only a few months ago. A friend gave me a pedicure as a gift and we went to one of the Chop Shops up on the Heights. If I'd known then that I would soon be doing them, I would have paid more attention. The Beauty Girls, of course, have been polishing their nails since the day they were conceived, so they're pros at it.

The color I pick for my own toes is a neutral, subdued coral and the Beauty Girls won't have any of it. They say it is just *too vanilla for words* and embarrassing. They say it is "*Fall for godssake*" and the season should be celebrated in style. They pick out a dark Fall Foliage Brown in honor of the season and put it on my toes. It is a beautiful deep eggplant color. When my toes are done, the BGs love it. They say it looks wicked slutty.

I just can't wrestle with the holding the toe and the bottle of polish all in the same hand and then the dipping and the fanning of the brush and the even stroking with the other. I am clumsy and awkward and I get polish all over everything...all over the bottle, all over the toes, all over the front of my lab coat, somehow in my bra and my hair. My class gives me the dubious honor of the Best Finger Painter in school. There are just some things I will not be doing in my Women's Health Spa...and pedicures is one of them.

On Friday we take our Anatomy and Physiology exam and we all pass, albeit some by the skin of our teeth, but the Beauty Girls all make it.

Friday 4:31 PM: "Let's Blow This Popsicle Stand!" someone yells as we all stampede out the door.

Week Six:

Want a Glass of Wine With That?

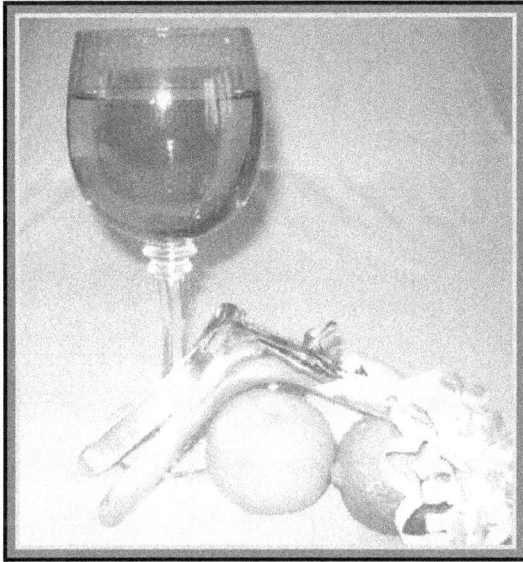

Still Life with Speculum

~)(~

Chapter 6

My face is starting to melt off my skull. By now we are getting different guinea pig facials about every other day and my skin is starting to wave a white hankie. As I said, I have never put anything more than Ivory Soap and Nivea on the old girl…and she is not tolerating it well. A couple of times my face has been "reactive" to unknown ingredients, that is to say the poor girl has blown up into a fiery red balloon and had to be packed in ice.

I know more about my skin "issues" than I had ever hoped to know. I have telangiectasia, erythema, hyperpigmentations…all really par for the course for "mature" skin. I have one large hyperpigmentation on my cheekbone where I was badly frost bitten once skiing a long time ago in the Rockies. Amazing what your skin will tell you.

In the beginning of this week, after yet another custom facial, we are introduced to Mineral Makeup, mainly because we all look like drowned rats after our facials, and this helps to make the service look more appealing. It really is miraculous stuff and I totally get into it. Mineral makeup is pure natural micronized mineral pigments with a built-in sun protection of SPF 15.

Now I know the secret of all the Senior Estheticians' look of serene, perfect beauty. When I put it on my own face, my skin looks flawless too. I love the stuff.

The Beauty Girls are surprised that I get into makeup but the truth is I've been wearing mineral makeup for over thirty years. I have brushed my face since the mid 1970's with "Indian Earth" which is some kind of mysterious dirt from Out West somewhere. It used to come in a little clay pot that would last for years. I have always credited Indian Earth as the reason why my skin is so healthy.

So this new Mineral Makeup is a beauty secret very familiar to me. I happily plaster everyone's face with Cool Beige and it instantly covers blemishes, discolorations and evens out skin tones. It hides a multitude of sins. This stuff is *the nuts*.

Toni is the first of the Beauty Girls to sign up for a Brazilian. I am ambivalent about Brazilians. After being a midwife for thirty years, I have seen my share of *WhoHa's* and I have seen the fads come and go. Some years it's in vogue to have a Mohawk or just a tiny little Landing Strip, some times it's the fashion to dye the *nether hair* a lush shiny color...or to grow out an unruly, untamed 70's bush.

Right now it's all the rage to sugar the Whole Enchilada...and that's what Toni has decided to do.

Toni is a striking young woman with porcelain skin and brooding dark eyes and long thick dark hair that is casually twisted up and tousled back with just the right amount of perfect messiness. This is the Beauty Girls' signature hairstyle.

A Senior is doing the service and Sophie is supervising the sugaring. I am doing a pedicure for an elderly woman who is talking to me non-stop. I have just spilled polish all over my glove and my glove is now stuck to the bottle and I can't get it off. I hear a bit of a ruckus coming from the Body Treatment rooms. The sound escalates until there is a piercing, blood-curdling scream. Toni. The scream rips through the Facial Room where the women freeze in mid-motion and it hits the Pedicure Room full force.

My client says, "Dear God! What was that?"

I decline to tell her that someone has just had all her pubic hair ripped out.

I say, "Well, I have no idea. Maybe someone stepped on a cat."

Sophie comes out of the Body Treatment room and her face is white with rage. She is livid that Toni was such a baby. Toni comes out of the room crying and slips quietly into the Ladies Room. I cannot shake the visual of her poor bald *WhoHa*. Sophie is exclaiming in a cluster of instructors; she is furious. This is the beginning of a long, rocky road between Toni and the instructors.

~)(~

This week we are studying Chemistry for Estheticians and now I am freaking out. Chemistry and I have never had a strong mutual attraction. Branches of Chemistry, Matter, Acidity and Alkalinity, Chemical Reactions, Chemistry as

Applied to Cosmeceuticals, Natural Ingredients. I know I need to know this, even if it is only to figure out the culprit ingredient that is making my face blow up so routinely. But instead what I find is...I am allergic to Chemistry.

Jett is a genius with product ingredients. She used to be a sales rep for a large line of botanical skin care products so she really knows her stuff. She is incredibly knowledgeable about the cause and effects of active ingredients, "Performance Ingredients." It seems overwhelming until I read somewhere about the possible carcinogenic-breast cancer link of certain preservatives, pabaparaben and methylparaben that are in almost everything. All of a sudden, I am real interested in researching this too.

I am watching Jett teach and I can tell she is deliberately leaving something out. Something that is important to her. She is very involved with the local organic farming community, green ecology, and preserving the Earth and our natural resources. What she really wants to teach the Beauty Girls is the *Mind-Body-Spirit* connection with the work we do. The potential deeper healing realm of our work; the realm of the soul. She is a Medicine Woman. I can tell she has been censored by the Convent and told to stick to the superficial, external physical domain of the epidermis. I can tell this frustrates her.

On Friday I take the Chemistry test and I pass...but just barely. It is a humbling experience. This esthetician idea is harder than I originally thought. This puts me in a very foul mood.

When I get home Tom is on the couch reading the paper. I know he's about to ask me, "What's for dinner?"

I'm just waiting for him to ask me that so I can bite his frickin' head off.

He looks up at me, grins and says, "Honey, can I get you a glass of wine?"

He grins wider and says, "Where would you like to go for dinner?" The boy is good. He's smooth. He's got great survival skills. He knows how to keep his unit intact.

Only four and a half months to go. Not sure today if I'm going to make it.

Week Seven:

Sperm Eyebrows

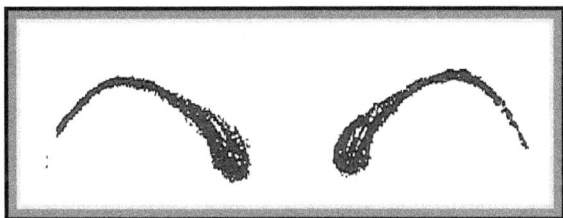

Classic Sperm Eyebrows

~)(~

Chapter 7

For months now, I have been watching the Seniors go back and forth to work out front in the clinic. I haven't even dared go out there yet to check it out. But this week is "Transition to Clinic" which means we are going to be slowly introduced to working out front with "real people." It seems mind-boggling to me that we are at this point in our training, because I still don't feel like I really have a clue yet as to what I am doing. I still feel awkward and stumbly...my classmates have begun to call me "Grace."

The first of the Beauty Girls chosen to work out front is Jacqueline. Jacqueline used to manage and oversee the entire dining room of a famous "old money" resort hotel up in the White Mountains. She is a very poised, regal young woman. She has streaked blond hair cut in a long stylish shag, large intense cat's eyes—a strange yellow brown color that gives her a compelling exotic look. Perfect eyeliner. Large smile. She walks with a very straight back, which I guess is my nice way of saying I think she may also be a tad of a control freak.

Jacqueline is instructed to do a facial on a paying customer. She swallows hard, straps on her fanny pack, and heads out front walking tall with her pert ponytail swaying back and forth. A true example of the image of the Perfect Esthetician. The other Beauty Girls jealously watch her leave us.

I, on the other hand, am the first chosen to cover the Front Desk because of my good "people skills." Great. Just what I signed up for…receptionist. For a while I see a definite pattern with the job assignments. The older, more mature women on the front desk, polished matronly smiles, "May I help you, dear?" contrasted to the young perky twenty-somethings bopping around doing the real services out front. When I mention my perception of this ageism, the Beauty Girls argue with me and tell me I'm high on crack.

~)(~

Mid-week I get a surreptitious email that our Midwives Insurance Equity Bill is going to be killed. I write a frantic email to all the members of the House Commerce Committee beseeching them to re-hear it. I explain that if this happens, all the freestanding birth centers in the state will be forced to close. The midwives will be driven out of business. The Chairman agrees to reconsider if I can make peace, somehow, with the insurance lobbyists and come up with language that works for both sides. Right. No problem. You kidding me? This is like getting the Bush Administration to embrace gay marriage. The Chair sets a date for a hearing in two weeks.

This week we learn lash and brow tinting and brow shaping. I am working with Lydia on this. Lydia is the "Woman of Indeterminate Age" who sat with me in the Hot

Flash Row on the first day of school. Lydia is a woman of many contradictions. I get the sense that she is a very intelligent, conscientious young woman yet she is covered with multiple facial piercings. A young woman of high moral standards and a gazillion tattoos. Lydia has decided she absolutely hates the Convent. She seems so sweet while at the same time muttering invectives under her breath: the "passive aggressiveness" of the Mother Superior is "such bullshit." She says the MS's approach is demeaning and belittling, and Lydia is becoming more pissed and more outspoken about this opinion as time goes on.

Lydia has enormous blue eyes, and the best thing is she has virgin eyebrows. She has thick dark brows that have never been plucked, tweezed, colored, penciled or messed with in any way. This is very unusual for a Beauty Girl. Most of the Beauteous Ones have tweezed their brows to a very fine line. This look is in vogue but I personally think this detracts a lot from the expressiveness the brows give the face. I am going to shape and color Lydia's virgin brows. She's nervous. It's her first time. I promise her I will make them perfect and not too thin.

All she says is, "Please don't give me Sperm Eyebrows."

We start brow sugaring by measuring and marking the landmarks of the brow itself. The inner brow, arch of the brow, outer landmark. We slather on a thin layer of sugar, just below the brow hairs, then take our little metal spatulas and pull the brow hairs we want to remove down into the sugar. This is a pretty precise technique. This way there is no chance of making a mistake and unintentionally ripping off part of the wanted brow. I know I am making Lydia's brow a fabulous shape. I like this. I feel confident. I *schwip! schwip!* and I think her brow is perfect. Lydia is looking more and more beauteous with every *schwip!*

Next is the lash and brow tinting. The color is vegetable dye; so theoretically, it is not dangerous to the eyes and reduces the need for mascara. For Lydia, I tint her eyelashes blue-black with a very subtle eyeliner just above the lashes. I do her brows dark blond but I do not leave it on very long. When I am done I hold up a mirror for her to see. She has been transformed from innocent, innocuous College Coed to sultry Vampy Beauty. She absolutely loves it.

When it's my turn, I trust Lydia completely. In my youth I used to have natural arched brows, but with the ravages of time they have become sparse and almost invisible. There really isn't anything to "shape" so Lydia just tints my lashes black and my brows brown. When she is done I look in the mirror and I can't believe my eyes. My face and my expression is so enlivened, my eyes so animated and naughty looking. Trampola! This stuff is so SASSY! I'm doing this every month like clockwork, come hell or high water.

~)(~

On Friday, I leave school early because I have set up a meeting with the lobbyists for the three major insurance carriers at a local watering hole. I sit waiting for them to show up and I am a tad nervous. This really is colluding with the enemy. They have lied and stalled and objected to everything they could think of to defeat our bill. All because insurance companies don't "like" insurance mandates. Well, *too bad*. Right now in New Hampshire, insured women are not able to give birth in birth centers and that is against their constitutional rights. I order a glass of Chardonnay to kill the coming pain.

The three women lobbyists arrive. One is tall and willowy and elegant. She is an attorney, the former insurance commissioner for the state and she is smart as hell. I respect her. She is impeccably and tastefully dressed. She reminds me of the Duchess of Windsor. To my relief, she orders a glass of wine as well…Merlot. I recognize right away that she is the Alpha-female.

The second lobbyist is a wiry, shorthaired redhead whose skin is very wrinkled and in dire need of help. It's embarrassing to admit that since I have been in the beauty biz, I notice women's skin very critically. I can be standing in the check-out line at the grocery store, look at a woman's brows and think, "Whoosh. If only I could get my hands on those unruly bad boys."

Anyway, the Redhead has always been cagey and I don't trust her as far as I can pee in the wind. She is a loose cannon.

The third lobbyist is short with a blond bob and she is also incredibly wrinkled. But her skin is sallow; it's not from sun damage. It's asphyxiated from years of smoking four packs a day. Her voice is gravelly and deep. She sits smoking, leaning away from us and blowing the smoke away over her shoulder. An overhead fan blows it right back in our faces. Great. She is the Poster Girl for Blue Cross/Blue Shield. She also orders a glass of wine to wash down her butts. I know deep down in her oxygen-deprived heart, she really likes me. But I also know she will follow suit with the Willowy One.

I explain to them the status of our bill and the implications for childbearing women in NH. In the NH Legislature, when a bill dies, it cannot be re-introduced for two years. The birth centers cannot survive that long without third party reimbursement. Within five minutes we come up with language that is satisfactory to both sides.

It's either the wine talking or my three new best friends, but either way, it's a bloody miracle. They agree to cover "state licensed facilities" only, no homebirths. I tell them that the state's midwives doing homebirths are going to think I sold them down the river, but I have been negotiating this for a long time and am politically savvy enough to know that this is a tremendous victory.

If only I can trust them to keep their word for two whole weeks.

And, frankly, I've lost all track of how much time I have been incarcerated in the Convent.

Week Eight:

Halloween and Shaman Smoke

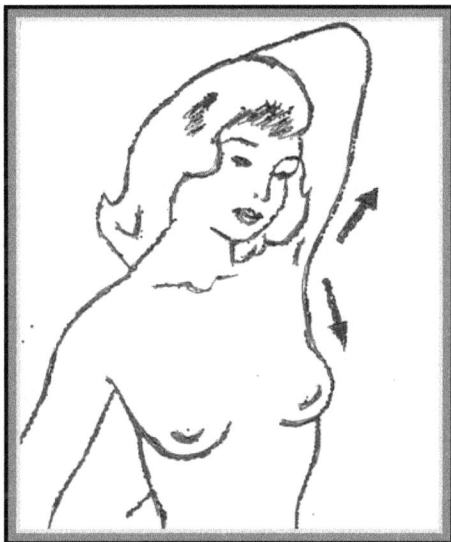

Underarms

~)(~

Chapter 8

The end of this week is Halloween. Halloween! I can't believe it. In Assembly, we are instructed by the Mother Superior to wear "Fantasy Makeup" on Friday for Halloween. She tells us to be creative, to "have fun with it." Somehow the word "fun" coming from her lips seems like an oxymoron. Yes, ma'am, alrighty then—we will have fun, *dammit*.

On Tuesday morning, we all go down into the bowels of the building to a pretty creepy basement room that is surrounded by mirrors on all four walls. We sit at stations and are instructed in the fine art and subtle nuances of professional makeup application. We are taught today by none other than the MS herself because she is considered the absolute Queen of Makeup.

The Mother Superior actually does know a lot and it's pretty fun and interesting, although, honestly, in my life I can't even imagine one case, unless it's in a morgue, where I will ever be using this knowledge. She shows us how to accentuate positive attributes with lighter colors and conceal negative features with darker shades. She is clearly in her element doing this stuff. We learn safe application of blush, eye shadow, eyeliner, mascara, eyebrow color, lip liner and lip color. Never in my life did I think I would be doing this.

When it comes time to do the eyebrow color, the MS uses me for the demonstration. Perhaps it's because my thinning brows need so much restoration and she can perform a miracle. I am sitting on a stool in the center of the brightly lit room with all the Beauty Girls standing around observing in their crisp white lab coats. It's like a scene straight out of the Fifties—or from Young Frankenstein. The MS demonstrates the skillful backward coloring stroke to fill in sparse patches with pencil for a natural look.

When I turn to look in the mirrors that surround me on all sides, I see an infinity of reflections of me with two huge black caterpillars over my eyes. Groucho Marx. I wriggle my eyebrows up and down and the caterpillars follow suit...up...down. All I need is a cigar. The BGs are trying to be serious but they cannot pull it off and burst into delighted squeals of laughter. Even the Mother S. herself cracks a slight hint of a smile and hands me a dampened gauze to exterminate the wayward caterpillars.

Some things are just not meant to be improved upon.

I am still a little shy about being out in the clinic. One day this week I am quietly walking out front through the facial

74

room. There is a woman lying on one of the tables with the heat mask on.

Her eyes follow me.

I can't tell if she's a student or a Real Person, so I politely say, "How you doing?"

She says, "*Waddup* yourself, you fat-ass cunt lips."

I say, "Oh, hi, Nikita. How the zits going, you WASP pizza face."

I do believe the girl may have Tourette's Syndrome.

For Halloween I decide to go as Bette. I ask Bette to get to school a little early so she can help do my face. I wear a black wig that is cut roughly in the shape of Bette's shag hair. She brings a razor and does a quick razor cut and spikes it to make it look identical to hers. She blacks my eyebrows, does purple eye shadow and scarlet lips. I have worn Bette-type glitzy earrings. We are in the bathroom and the Assembly has started. I put on raspberry colored glasses like hers and we collapse in hysteria. It's a little frightening. We look like clones. Tweedle Dee and Tweedle Dum.

I put her nametag ~Bette~ on my lab coat.

We walk out of the bathroom into the Assembly as the MS is speaking. Even she cracks up…we bring down the house. Nice. Nicely done. Now I am to be Bette for the entire day. I look in the mirrors that surround the entire room and realize I look like a man. I look like a man dressed in drag trying to impersonate a glamorous middle-aged woman. With the spiked black hair and the black eyebrows, I could be an out-of-work cross dresser trying to do Liza Minneli. God. It's going to be a long day in this get-up.

In the morning I am assigned to sugar a new client's bikini line. I know I look so much like a transvestite it's scary. When I meet her, I shake her hand and pitch my voice low like a man's and say, "So, you want to be sugared, *Shuga*?"

She looks horrified and turns like she is about to flee out the door. I laugh and apologize and say that I am in costume. She is not amused. She obviously thinks I am very sketchy.

By late afternoon my eyebrows have been smudged and are seriously starting to head south. I am wearing one of our horrible stretchy white hair bonnets pretending I am a Lunch Lady. I am walking around with my black hair and black eyebrows and the hair bonnet, growling, "You want mashed potatoes with that?"

~)(~

I am assigned at the end of the day to do pedicures for walk-ins. I keep my costume on, still wearing the Lunch Lady bonnet. I am polishing the woman's toes for her first time ever. She is a quiet, reserved woman. I am making flip conversation with her. I ask her where she works. She responds that she works in the cafeteria at the Technical Institute.

Omigod. She IS a lunch lady. I feel really bad and discreetly slip my bonnet into my pocket. What a dipshit I am.

Yet for some reason unbeknownst to humankind, my flipness continues uncensored. The woman has a huge divet in her leg.

As I am massaging her limb, I point to the crater and ask, "What'd an alligator get you?"

She responds quietly, "No, I had a bad skin cancer."

OK...WHY would I ever even ask something like that? It obviously couldn't have been anything good. Jesus...what a *jackass*.

I point to my nametag that says ~Bette~.

The hands-down winner of this year's Fantasy Makeup Contest, in my opinion, is the young instructor, Delores. Delores supervises the scheduling and the functioning of the clinic. We weren't really involved with Delores until we graduated to "the front" but by now I've come to understand she really is the intercellular cement that holds the whole scene together...seemingly seamlessly. I'm beginning to realize the place would fall apart without her. She is young in years, but ageless in her dedication to the running and direction of the Convent...sometimes ruthlessly so. She takes her job very seriously.

Delores is pretty with intense blue eyes and jet-black hair. Her lower back is embellished with a huge tat of *Kwuan Yin*, the Goddess of Compassion. Today Delores's fantasy face is astounding. She has painted one side of her face a fire opal white, and the other side a luminescent turquoise, the colors found in abalone shells. Her face is decorated with primitive tribal markings. She is wearing a headdress of bright blue and green Macaw feathers that go straight up from her crown. She has transformed herself into an Aztec priestess. The result is incredibly powerful and breathtaking.

In the late afternoon, Delores, Merrill and I are in the front pedicure room and it is quiet. Delores is doing Merrill's makeup because Merrill and her metro-sexual boyfriend, Todd, are going to a costume party later in the evening. Delores has a great palette to work with...Merrill is arguably the most beautiful of all the Beauty Girls. She is drop-dead gorgeous in the classic Town and Country sense of perfection, complete with requisite giant diamond stud earrings.

Merrill is going to a Halloween party costumed as a brick house. Truly. She is wearing a dress that is printed as a brick house. The brick house has windows that open at the boobs and a door at the pubes that opens and has a little cat in the doorway. A cute little pussy...cat. Her boyfriend is going as a brick layer. He is carrying a trowel and wearing a jumpsuit that says "Dick Fitzwell Bricklayers".

Delores has decided to do Merrill's face as "Smoke", as in smoke coming out of the chimney of the brick house. I am sprawled across a pedi chair silently watching them. I am mesmerized witnessing this transformation. I have never expected makeup to be so fascinating. I am watching Delores with her Aztec Priestess face and her parrot feather headdress changing Merrill's face into Smoke.

The reality begins to blur for me. I see Delores initiating a young priestess in a Rite of Passage. I am in a jungle somewhere watching a Shaman Woman transform the younger one by painting her face. Painting her in the Ancient Way that only the tribe knows. The power of the painting to shape shift reality. The power to prepare the younger one to face what is ahead for her. The power to protect her and keep her strong. Now I understand the roots to all this. As Delores paints, Merrill changes.

Delores's hand is steady and sure. She knows what she is doing. Merrill's face is transformed into light and dark curling wisps of smoke. Smoke curling around and through her eyes. Smoldering wisps trailing up through her hairline. The beauty and the power of the smoke to protect and guide her, to transform the young initiate to bravely walk the path ahead for her.

When Delores is done, Merrill turns to me and she is She Who Is Smoke. I cannot speak. Then someone comes in to the pedi room and the spell is broken.

What I *first* think is, Whew. I got to lay off the caffeine.

What I *really* think is, I am so honored to be with these guys.

Time to go home and get ready for Trick-or-Treaters, but first I have to buy a bunch of little cans of Spam for them.

Week Nine:

Hooters Airline

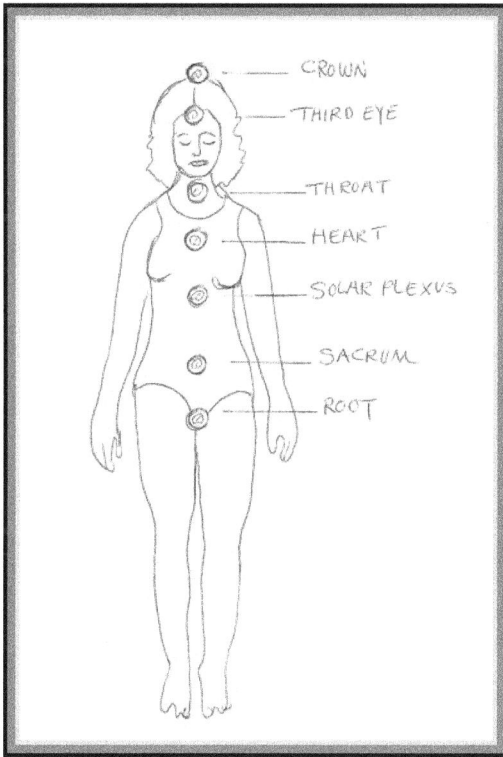

The Seven Major Chakras

~)(~

Chapter 9

Vivienne's eyebrows have come down a couple of stories. She's trying to let them grow in but every time she comes back from a weekend, they're gone again. She says she's addicted to tweezing them and can't stop. She needs to go to a twelve-step program for this nervous habit, Pluckers Anonymous.

Watching her pencil them on is an art form in itself. She measures meticulously and outlines, then fills in with flawless black pencil. She is incredibly good at this. Still when she looks at you with those arched brows, it looks like she's perpetually saying, "Oh really?"

She looks like the Grouchy Ladybug.

At the beginning of this week we are assigned a partner to role-play "Needs Assessments." I hate role-playing; it always seems so forced, so fake.

My assigned partner is Angel. Angel was in the class ahead of us but she is the only one continuing on for the Advanced Esthetics Program, so she has been adopted into our class. Angel is a strange Goth kid. She is short but wears shoes that have a six-inch heel so she seems taller. She also seems a lot older than she really is…she is fresh out of high school. She has long straight dark hair and wears a ton of makeup, thick black eyeliner. The effect is close to Morticia from the Addams Family.

We are supposed to be interviewing each other about "When was the last time you loved the look and feel of your skin?" I hate this fakeness, so I say that I loved my skin this morning. Angel announces that she won't be doing any of this in real life because she hates people and doesn't give a rat's ass whether they like their skin or not. All she wants to do is hair removal. I suggest that perhaps she is in the wrong profession with that attitude. She is sulky and petulant and just sits there toying with her jade pierced tongue stud and twisting her hair around her finger. The hour is excruciating. This puts me in a very foul mood.

There is a new class that has started this week. I guess that means we are now promoted to Juniors. Some of the Seniors are graduating as they hit the 600 hour mark. The day they leave they have a "Day of Beauty" which means they can have all the personal services they want before they are out the door. They have pedicures, facials, various sugarings and body treatments from us...then we never see them again. They vanish out into the Real World.

The new class is small. There are only five of them, two Older Women around my age and three young twenty-somethings. They are very shy and quiet. They slink around timidly and whisper inaudibly amongst themselves at lunch. It never occurs to me that my class is so insanely loud that we intimidate the hell out of them. We sit all day in the "study hall" staring at our textbook, Milady. (I'm completely serious, that's the name of our educational text. MILADY. *Jasus.*) We sit for hours on end while the new class is stuck in the classroom all day with Sophie. For some reason I resent the new class. I acknowledge that this is a very immature reaction but for some reason they bug the snot out of me.

Something is going on this week...something bad. Everyone is having meltdowns of one kind or another. Bette cries all through lunch after recounting a recent painful event. Mary sobs uncontrollably after a shitty experience with a service. Toni weeps about a bad breakup with her boyfriend and has to leave and go home. Jacqueline has rearranged our tables so we can study better; Angel disapproves and puts them back the way they were. Jacqueline bursts into tears and something about this sets my midwife antennae on alert. Hmmm...

Personally, I feel like I am crawling out of my skin with boredom. I feel like we are all just festering here, biding our time until we are paroled. Everyone is bitchy and raggy and having an absolutely *suckass* week.

I am working the front desk in the afternoon and I am bored. The front desk is either mind-numbingly dull or is a frenzy of hectic activity. The phone rings and I answer the way we have been instructed to.

"Esthetics Institute. This is Carol. How may I help you?"

It is a voice I recognize but the woman won't talk to me; she asks to speak to an instructor. The instructor comes out and pencils in the woman's name for a brow shape and tint for this afternoon. The woman is a former best friend of mine who has told people that she is embarrassed that I am here. She is mortified that I am in beauty school, yet she is still coming here for her brows. I am pissed.

Pearl has been assigned to take care of her.

I go out back where all the Beauty Girls are sitting around gossiping and eating pounds of chocolate.

I say, "Pearl, you have a brow this afternoon. The client is an ex-friend of mine; she's a dirty blond. I'll pay you $50 bucks if you make a "mistake" and tint her brows jet black."

Pearl's eyes slowly grow wide as what I have said sinks in.

She says, "You mean you want me to make a mithtake on purpoth?" She is incredulous. "That'th juth not ethical," she lisps. She stomps out of the room with her fanny-pack jouncing.

The Beauty Girls watch her walk away.

"Fucking idiot," Toni says. "I'd have done it in a heartbeat."

The tension builds all week until it is almost palpable. There is something seriously wrong with all of us. It's to the point where I wonder if it could be a good old fashioned case of Mass Hysteria. We can smell it in the air. The Ladies Room is just nasty with the rank smell. No amount of Febreze can disguise the odor. Then I recognize it…Hormones! Estrogen!

WARNING! WE ARE ALL SUFFERING FROM SEVERE ESTROGEN POISONING!

There are just *way* too many Alpha Bitches in this place.

~)(~

In the middle of the week is the legislative hearing for the Midwives Insurance Equity Bill. I miss school Wednesday morning and go to the State House to represent the New Hampshire Midwives Association. When I arrive the three insurance lobbyists are there sitting in the front row.

I sit down with them. The Chair raises her eyebrow in surprise. She asks if we have come to a resolve and I say "Yes."

The Lobbyists hand her a copy of the proposed Amendment. She asks me if I approve. I take a look at it and see a clause snuck in there that would prohibit our inclusion. I start to lose my temper, but the Willowy One rephrases it to say "if applicable," which everyone agrees to. Then I start to grin because this, of course, renders it meaningless. Now it is open to very broad interpretation. The Willowy One winks at me; she knows we have just won.

Our bill is voted on and approved unanimously. It is to be on the House Consent Calendar which means it won't be debated on the floor. It's a done deal. I can't believe it. After thirty years of jousting against the Windmill...I have won. I have beaten the Machine. This is my swan song (or so I think at the time.) How we did it I don't know. Maybe it was the marriage of Chardonnay and Merlot, but such are the mysterious workings of This Great Democracy of Ours. New Hampshire—"Live Free or Die," you got to love it.

After the hearing, everyone is clapping me on my back congratulating me. They know how hard the Midwives have worked for this. This was a great grassroots campaign. I think everyone is glad that it is finally over. I know some Reps are actually very surprised that we have pulled off this victory. My old friend Crow, who was our prime sponsor, gives me a huge bear hug and calls me "Dominatrix Quixote." This puts me in a very good mood.

~)(~

On Thursday morning Jacqueline whispers that she wants to talk to me. We step outside on the stoop to the backdoor. Her eyes are dancing. She grabs me by my shoulders and says, "I'm pregnant! I did a pregnancy test this morning and it was positive! I haven't even told my husband yet. This is so unreal...I'm pregnant! God! This is the first time we've even tried...and it worked! I'm so excited!"

I thought as much.

I say, "Wow! Congratulations, sweetie! That's great news!"

She says, "Please don't tell the others just yet. I want to tell my husband first."

I say of course, absolutely, I understand.

I go back in and write on a little post-it note, *Jacqueline is pregnant!* and slip it to Bette and Mary.

This week we begin to learn the various types of Body Treatments. I like these services. I am definitely going to offer them in my Natural Woman's Holistic Health Spa. We learn Full Body Exfoliation, Lymphatic Drainage and Dry Brushing.

On Friday we are doing a Detoxifying Herbal Wrap which helps to eliminate toxins from the body. Muslin sheets are soaked in an infusion of Lavender, Calendula Petals, Clove, Eucalyptus, Ginger Root and Rosemary to draw out impurities. The sheets are extremely hot and aromatic.

We take turns "cocooning" each other in the wet, hot sheets. I am working with Vivienne. It seems she and I get paired up a lot together. I like Vivienne because she has such an intelligent, quick humor. Vivienne says her claim to fame in high school was that she was the first person to get suspended three years in a row.

We take turns exfoliating each other's body with either a dry brush or rough gloves. Then we get naked on top of the herbal sheets that are as hot as we can tolerate. This is wrapped with a plastic sheet, then with a heated blanket. We are left to sweat it out for 20 minutes.

I go first and Vivienne wraps me tightly. She tells me to "relax and enjoy" and then leaves the darkened little treatment room.

I think, "God, if I detox all the wine I drank last night I'm going to be peeing for a month." Slowly I start to get inordinately hot. Hot flash. Then my heart skips a beat and then it starts beating very fast. My breathing gets jagged. My heart is crashing against my chest. I am too tightly wrapped and I can't get out. I am like a mummy.

Help!

I start to wriggle and twist to try to get unwrapped. I am claustrophobic. My lips are going numb. My arms are pinned against my sides. My fingers are tingling. Blind Panic. Must get my arms out. I am making a strange squeaking noise.

Help!

I try to lift my head. Impossible. I bend my knees. Then straighten my legs out. Bend again. I must look like a frenzied Inch Worm. I am thrashing around frantically. I flop on my side. Finally, somehow I get my arms free. Once my hands are loose I calm down.

Vivienne comes back in and says, "How you doing?"

I say, "Oh fine. *Fine*. Next time might want to leave the arms out though."

She says, "Man, you are *really sweating*."

Vivienne has an awesome tattoo on her lower back. It is a large Celtic cross with "Thy Will Be Done" right above her butt crack. Her family crest. When it is her turn and she is cocooned, I decide to do some energy work for her—Chakra Balancing.

I start at her head, rocking her gently down her right side to her feet. At her feet I do a little Reflexology. Then I move slowly back up to her head with my hands gently rocking at each of the seven Chakra points. Vivienne makes a weird sound. The sound gets louder. Vivienne is sound asleep and snoring.

~)(~

Things at the Convent have gotten much better now that everyone is running around half naked again. Laughing faces, slender bodies, perky breasts, sugared *WhoHa's*, tattooed backsides, navels pierced with diamond belly rings. Things are back to normal.

On Friday we are finally released from the Convent for the weekend. The Beauty Girls are walking en masse down the sidewalk to our cars, towing our wheeled-rolling suitcases behind us.

An attractive man steps out of Gibson's bookstore and gives us the Kooky Eye.

"Have a nice trip ladies," he says.

Merrill turns and flashes him a blinding smile.

"Excuse me, sir. We're flight attendants for Hooters Airline. Are you a Frequent Flyer? Perhaps you can tell us the way to Manchester Airport?"

We all howl. *Damn*, that girl's got ovaries.

The Beauty Girls strike again.

Bless their little Black Hearts.

Week Ten:

Burn, Baby, Burn

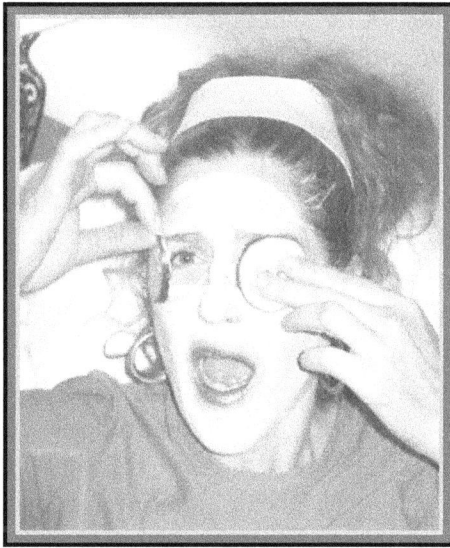

HOLY BAD ACID DRIP!

~)(~

Chapter 10

I am halfway through the Program. I can't believe it. Half way to Freedom! The rest of my class is going to continue on for the Advanced Clinical Esthetics Program, which is an additional 300 hours. As much as I truly love these guys, I just want to get my license and get out of here and start working. The thought of being in here for an extra three months with the Mother Superior makes my nose start to bleed.

Shrimpy has been missing a lot of school. I am worried about her. When she does show up she looks pale and drawn and upset. Her lab coat is wrinkled and looks like "a dog's breakfast" as my grandmother used to say. I know Shrimpy has the worst schedule of all the Beauty Girls. She works the graveyard shift at Bickford's from 11:00 PM to 6:00 AM and then she drags ass to school for 8:30. She has been arriving late or sometimes not at all.

I am concerned that maybe her live-in boyfriend is being abusive to her...or she is coming to school baked...or doing drugs. Something is definitely amiss. All I can do is wait patiently and hope that she'll talk to me when she's ready. She is such a sweet kid. She's knows I'm open for conversation with her at any time.

This week we learn Alpha Hydroxy Acid Peels. According to Milady, "AHAs theoretically normalize the Stratum Corneum by reducing its thickness through deep exfoliation. These peels create a more compact structure in the skin by increasing dermal thickness due to increased hydration and a normalization of skin functions. They increase skin hydration due to the natural moisturizing properties of AHAs by activating hyaluronic acid which, in turn, will retain a greater amount of moisture in the skin."

We memorize Glycolic Acid from Sugar Cane, Lactic Acid from Sour Milk, Tartaric Acid from Sour Grapes, Citric Acid from Fruit, Malic Acid from Rotting Apples.

We practice on mannequins until we get the drill down pat. Set timer for 60 seconds. Wipe acid on face quickly, making sure not to overlap. When timer dings, grab 4 x 4s that have been soaking in ice water to cool down burn. Wipe. Ice. Wipe. Ice. Wipe. Then Aloe Vera with cortisone cream to lessen the pain. The instructors hover nervously. I envision clients screaming in agony with permanently scarred, disfigured faces. I wonder what my liability is. I realize that I let my malpractice insurance lapse. I think the whole thing is traumatic.

For the first Real Peel I am paired with Nikita. We are using Lactic Acid 3.0. It smells suspiciously like baby spit-up. I go first. I am a little tense because Bette says her face hurt like hell and I know my skin is much more reactive than hers. But when Nikita puts the Lactic Acid on me, to my relief, I only feel a slight stinging sensation.

Bette is doing a custom facial for a Real Person on the table next to us. I know she is observing the whole thing out of the corner of her eye.

The tables are turned and I am doing Nikita's AHA. I am nervous because I know what a spaz I can be sometimes. Nikita herself is oddly silent, probably a good indication that she is truly terrified. I set my timer and Jett pours the acid on my outstretched gauzed fingers.

I swipe, swipe, swipe Nikita's trusting, upturned face.

Jett is like a condor, waiting.

She says urgently, "Quickly! Quickly! Quickly!"

This is freaking me out.

Jett points and says, "It's pooling. It's dripping into her eye!"

I say, "Jesus Christ!" I reach for the gauze that is on my station to wipe Nikita's eye.

Jett grabs my wrist roughly and squeezes her nails in.

Jett says, "Stop! That's the gauze with the acid on it!"

I yell, "HOLY BAD ACID DRIP!" as I realize in horror that I almost wiped Nikita's eye with acid soaked gauze.

Jett growls, "Watch your mouth" and nods to the Real Person on the next table.

I say, "I can't help it. It's her fault." I point to Nikita. "*Tourette's*. It's highly contagious."

I hear the neighboring Real Person whisper to Bette, "Good God, who is that student? I want to be sure I never get her."

Bette says, "Grace. Her name is Grace."

Jett shakes her head, sighs deeply and walks away.

Nikita relaxes. She looks up at me with her perfectly acid-polished face.

"Wow. What an awesome vid. I was just eye-level with Jett's camel toe. Total *beef curtains*!"

Note to Self: Always dispose of acid soaked gauze.

Other Note to Self: Look in Want Ads. May not be cut out for this work.

My own face is looking pretty good. Friends are actually commenting on how fabulous my skin looks. I have to admit my skin really does feel better than it has in years. It could be the facials I am getting every five minutes, but I attribute the marked improvement to the miracle of Vitamin C. Vitamin C, or Ascorbic Acid, is an essential antioxidant needed for proper repair of skin cells and healing of tissues. We are told it plays an important role in fighting the aging process and promotes collagen production in the dermal layer, keeping the skin healthy and firm. After being a cranky skeptic...I'm a believer.

As Jett says, Vitamin C "Whitens, Tightens and Brightens." It really does. I notice the difference immediately. It makes mature skin radiant.

Vitamin C has become my beauty secret. I go crazy with it in my daily routine. I use Vibran-C Mist which is a spray toner, then several squirts of Complex C Serum, a Vitamin C concentrate that costs an arm and a leg, then slather on Complex C moisturizer. I still have Scrotum Eyes, but my skin looks marvelous.

One day as I walk past the front desk the phone rings. Pearl is manning the front desk and she answers the way we have been instructed to. I swear I hear her say with her little lisp;

"Pathetic Insthitute. Thith ith Pearl. How may I help you?"

PATHETIC Institute?!? Judas Priest.

"Pearly, Pearly, darling girl…it sounds for all the world like you're saying 'Pathetic' Institute."

"Really?" She does her little hiccupy laugh and flutters her unbearably long lashes.

"It's Esth…say Esth." I coach her.

"Ehth…I can't. Ith too hard."

Omigod.

~)(~

Toward the end of the week I am sitting in the far pedi chair getting my "Personal Service" of the week, a Classic Pedicure. By now I have fully graduated to slutty colors, my current fave being a dark berry color called "Berry Hard." I am flipping through a trade magazine, SKIN INC. and semi-snoozing. A few other Beauty Girls are also getting pedicures. They are sitting in the other chairs gossiping viciously about a student in the class ahead of us who they suspect is doing drugs.

Across the room, Goth Angel is taking care of an elderly gentleman named Horace. She is being very tender and gentle with him. It is his first time here. Apparently his feet have been bothering him terribly, so he wandered in for a good soak and a trim. His feet are very gnarled and disfigured from age. They do look uncomfortable. Angel asks him if the temperature of the foot soak is OK. She is being very caring and careful with Horace.

The Beauty Girls are discussing what kind of drugs could cause the jitteriness and shakiness in the Senior they are gossiping about. One of the BGs says she thinks it looks like an extreme crystal meth habit. They wonder if the Mother Superior is aware of this student's deteriorating condition. They wonder if the Senior is smoking it when she goes out in the alleyway for her numerous breaks. They are really trash-talking this student.

Angel is massaging Horace's calloused feet. Suddenly she whips around with her long black hair flying and confronts the Beauty Girls.

She says forcefully, "Stop it you guys! I mean it! Stop it right now!"

She is embarrassed and is protecting her client.

The Beauty Girls roll their eyes and look at each other like "Whatever" but they do fall silent.

For a kid who claims she hates people, Angel is being pretty wonderful with this old man. I think there may be more to this kid than meets the eye.

~)(~

On Friday, we learn another full body treatment, the "Salt Glow Body Polish," which uses large crystals of sea salt mixed with jojoba oil as an extreme exfoliant. Even though it is quite messy, I like this treatment a lot. It leaves your skin feeling zippy and incredibly soft.

I am telling Bette about trying to give Tom a "Salt Glow Body Polish" over the weekend and what a total pain in the ass he is because all he does is ask when is his Happy Ending.

Bette growls and says, yeah, when her husband acts up like that, she tells him he's not even going to get a Happy Beginning.

Ten more weeks to go… C. U. Next Tuesday…as the Beauty Girls always say.

Week Eleven:

La Femme Nikita's Broken Nose

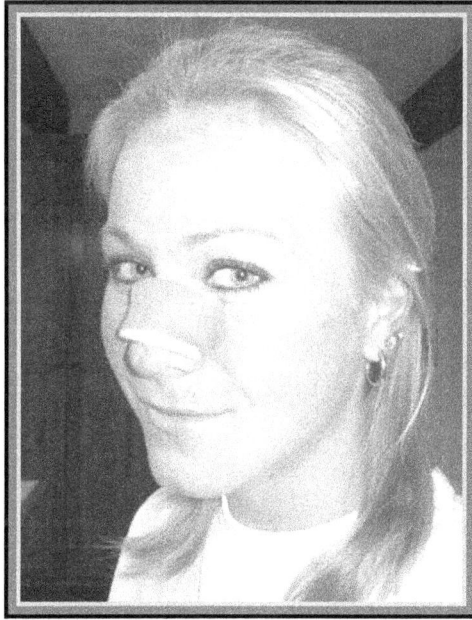

La Femme Nikita

~)(~

Chapter 11

We are sitting in the upstairs classroom supposedly studying Product Ingredients but mostly the Beauty Girls are recapping their favorite events from the past weekend.

I find this room to be strangely unsettling. Again it is garishly lit, but it has these funky little windows that slide open and overlook the big "study hall" below. I can see the new students all huddled at their tables down below us. Sometimes I see the Mother Superior up here looking down, watching us. This architecture is bizarre. Maybe it was a Reformatory Ward for Wayward Girls.

I look down the table to Nikita, who is strangely quiet. I'm thinking she's probably too hung over to participate in the fray. She looks terrible, actually. I look closer and realize she has two enormous black eyes. What the hell? Two huge purple-black shiners and it looks to me like her nose is crooked. Jesus. I'm hoping her boyfriend isn't responsible for this. I move over to sit next to her.

"What's going on, La Femme Nikita?"

Nikita looks at me and her eyes cross as she tries to focus over her swollen lopsided nose.

"My frickin' nose is killing me! I was snowboarding at Sunday River this weekend with a bunch of my friends. Maybe I was a little buzzed."

"A little buzzed?"

"OK. I was a *lot* buzzed and I caught my mother-fucking edge and did a fucking face plant right in this ice-encrusted snow. There was blood everywhere. My nose swelled up to the size of a football. I was seeing stars. I had to drink a bunch of Suffering Bastards to kill the pain. It's kind of better now."

I look closely. Nikita has broken her nose. Nikita has broken her nose snowboarding and she has toughed it out. What a scrappy kid.

I laugh. "Oh god, Nik, you Wild Thang. Mind if I take a look?"

I put my fingers on both sides of her nose and gently feel around. I palpate the bridge of her nose where the lump is. I can definitely feel the cartilage protruding out to one side. It is very floppy and moveable. I press a little firmer on the right side until I have a purchase on the break then I press hard and I feel it snap back in place with a loud crunch.

Nikita screams. "OWWWWWW! Holy Fuck You Ho Bag Bitch! What the Fuck?! Peace Out Bitch! Jesus Fucking Christ...chillax!"

Her eyes are tearing.

I laugh. Nikita's mouth sounds like she should be a contestant on the Jerry Springer Show. The White Trash litany; "Holy bleep You Ho Bag bleep! What the bleep?! Peace Out bleep! Bleep bleep bleep...chillax!" Right?

"You girls pipe down! What the hell is going on up there?" The Mother Super herself yells.

Ruh-roh. The funky little windows are open. Shit.

I reply, "Nothing! We're good. It's all good. Just doing a minor little nose job. Nothing to worry about."

Nikita...Nikita...Nikita. The Rebel Without a Clue.

In a week, the bruises around Nikita's eyes change from blue-black to a colorful yellow green with a hint of violet. Festive Easter colors. The swelling in her nose is reduced considerably. She no longer looks cross-eyed. She's beginning to look like Barbie again. Yep. Evil blue-eyed Barbie from Hell.

Toni has been butting heads with the instructors all along. Why she bothers to take this on I don't know, some kind of immature power struggle I guess. Challenge Authority. It's bad chemistry. She is constantly complaining about how mean they are to her. Sometimes her whining gets irritating but I have to agree that the instructors do seem to single her out and pick on her. She is always in tears but she won't back down.

This week she is fighting with them about her fingernails. She has on acrylic French Manicured fake nails that the instructors say are too long to wear out in the Clinic. Toni goes out to do a service with the nails on anyway...and gets canned from the floor. She is replaced with another student. Jett is screaming at her. Jett tells her to file them down before she claws someone by accident. Toni screams back that she has already filed them down…a couple of times. It's a bad scene. The Beauty Girls all hide behind their Miladys pretending not to notice. Holy Crap.

In Assembly the next morning, the instructors do a passive-aggressive lecture about acrylic nails and how unsanitary they are when doing services. It's pretty brutal. Everyone knows they are talking about Toni but they never divulge names. They say that fake nails can harbor the microorganisms that cause Staph infections. This is a danger to our clients. I find this interesting since we always wear gloves for all of our services.

Toni has tears streaming down her face. She says, "I hate this place" as she walks out the door.

In class, in the weird upstairs classroom, Jett is quizzing us with vocabulary words. The push is on to get us familiar with technical terms so we will score well on the State Boards. The school prides itself in a 93% pass rate for graduates of the Institute. They don't want our class to damage their good reputation. Sometimes I think they think the September class is a bunch of knuckleheads.

Pearl is sitting off by herself. Her hair is pulled back and up in a tight topknot. She has a very high forehead. Her skin is glowing pale and luminescent. Her enormous eyes are vacant and staring. She is wearing a gorgeous white leather jacket with a white fur collar. The child is pristine. She looks for all the world like a character out of Dr. Zhivago. I can just picture snowflakes on her long lashes. She catches me looking at her and gives me a big vacuous smile.

Jett calls out, "Ladies, what is Cataphoresis?"
The entire class is silent and rustles nervously.
Pearl answers, "That's the protheth of uthing galvanic current from the pothitive to the negative pole."

I think, "WHOA!" The Pearlster has really been studying her stuff.

Jett continues, "What is Catabolism?"

Stone cold silence from all of us.

Pearl answers again, "That's the phathe of breaking down complexth compounds rethulting in the releathe of energy."

Everyone looks at her in shock.

Pearl is a sandwich girl at Subway and she wants out of there. Pearl dreams of being an esthetician in the spa at the prestigious Wentworth-By-The-Sea resort hotel on the New Hampshire coast. Pearl wants this more than anything. She sits quietly studying and highlighting her Milady textbook 24/7. Pearl is working her ass off to get there.

At the end of the week we learn the Algae~Seaweed Wrap. This is a Full Body Treatment that detoxifies and re-mineralizes the skin with warm, protein-rich sea algae. This is another "cocooning" wrap that allows the sea algae's iodine, vitamins and minerals to penetrate the body. This treatment leaves the skin feeling amazing and it's my favorite wrap.

It's my favorite…except for the smell. The sea algae smells like dead lobsters. Seriously, it smells like polluted Low Tide. A lot of estheticians add drops of Essential Oil of Lavender to disguise the dead lobster smell, but I rather like it. I grew up on the Coast of Maine and my ancestors had a lobster pound. One of my fondest memories as a child is of my Grandfather chasing us around the dining table with a huge lobster claw stuck on his nose and the antennae sticking down from his lips, making the sound of a demented lobster. The smell of decomposing seafood always makes me nostalgic.

This day I am working with the regal Jacqueline and she is doing a Dead Lobster Wrap for me. I have forgotten, actually, that she is pregnant. Great midwife. I have been exfoliated and brushed and am lying on top of a plastic sheet. Jacqueline begins coating my back with the thick green algae on a camelhair paintbrush. It feels slimy. The algae smells particularly ripe today.

I am starting to drift off when I hear a gagging sound. Uh oh. Now I remember. My eyes fly open in time to see Jacqueline's shoulders heave. She leaps up from her stool and lunges toward the wastebasket in the corner of the room. She drops to her knees and buries her head in the trash liner and wretches violently. Poor kid. The low tide smell has really found its mark.

Ah, pregnancy. The Great Equalizer. She stands up and blows her nose. I hand her my cup of water.

"I'm sorry Sweetie," I say. "This nausea will only last for a few more weeks. It gets much better after you're past your first trimester. I promise."

"This whole thing is so humbling." She wipes her mouth. "But I'm going to do whatever it takes. I am so in awe that I have a whole new person growing in my belly!"

What a beautiful, beautiful woman.

I ask Bette to tint my eyebrows and lashes for the upcoming weekend. I'm feeling a little spunky and want to impress Tom. Bette and I are screwing around and gossiping as she tints. Unfortunately, the colors get reversed and she dyes my lashes light brown and my brows jet-black. My eyebrows are thick black smudges. I look like Groucho Marx's twin sister. "Say the magic woid and you win the prize." Dang. Not exactly the look I was going for.

Tom and I go out for drinks and dinner and he doesn't notice or say a thing about my new Joan Crawford imitation all evening.

The next morning when we wake with the sun coming in through our bedroom window, Tom rolls over and opens his sleepy eyes. His head snaps up as he looks at me and he screams, "ARRHHH!"

When he stops hyperventilating and has regained his composure, he says, "Jesus, honey, you scared me. This is like waking up in bed with Fred Flintstone."

So much for spunky.

I wiggle my eyebrows in a lame come-hither attempt. "Yabba dabba do?"

Week Twelve:

Amazing Grace

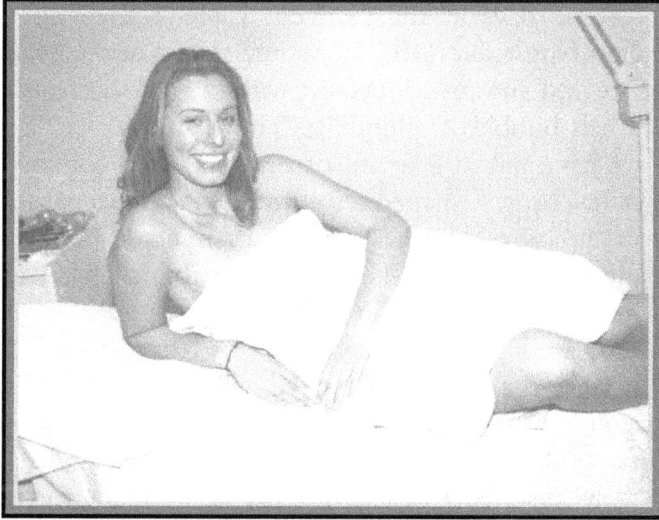

~)(~

Chapter 12

The end of this week is Thanksgiving. Thank the Holy Mother. I'm going to take a couple of days off because Tom's whole French Canadian family is coming to our house for Thanksgiving dinner. Tom's parents and all his older brothers and their families. We're going to cook two turkeys, one traditional roasted and one deep-fried in the Rocket Launcher. His family is great. They're always loud and funny and wholesome in a quirky way. Mostly we eat too much, drink too much, get tryptophan poisoning, take turns napping on the couch and then play cut-throat board games like Pictionary.

Some days at the Convent I feel really "on"...and some days I am really "off." For some reason in the beginning of this week, I am not connecting with the tasks at hand at all. I am "a half-bubble off plumb" as Tom says.

I have talked a friend of my son's into coming in to get her eyebrows shaped and tinted. She needs it. Her eyebrows are unruly bushes that need taming desperately. She has wandering hairs that stick out about an inch. They almost block her vision. She has Einstein eyebrows.

Sugar is pretty finicky stuff. You have to do all the steps in just the right order or it won't work at all. First cleanse with antimicrobial soap, then dry and sprinkle with a corn starch-like powder—'Pre-Epilation Product'. It has to be completely absolutely dry or it's just a wasted effort. I am working with my son's friend to conquer her disorderly brows and I do all the steps required:

I sanitize the area with the soap.

I sprinkle with powder to dry the area, use a Q-tip to smooth it out.

I scoop out some warm sugar from the sugar pot with my little spatula and coat it on the back of my glove. This will be my palette.

I apply an even, thin layer of sugar under the brow in the direction of hair growth.

I pull all the Bad Boys that I want to remove down into the sugar.

I smooth the little Pellon fabric strip over the sugar, warm it up.

I hold the eyebrow skin taut.

I *Schwip!* pull the fabric in the opposite direction of hair growth....and nothing happens. Nothing. *Nada.* All the renegade hairs are still there.

Damn.

I repeat the process.

Same thing. Nothing.

What the…?!?

I do this several more times. Not one hair leaves its mooring.

I am getting very frustrated. Needless to say, so is my young friend who has been bracing herself for orbital pain each time.

She says, "Umm…is there a problem here?"

What can I say? Every time I *Schwip!* the offending hairs are all still there…mocking me.

I am about to throw in the towel when I discover my mistake.

I have inadvertently grabbed Jojoba Oil instead of the Soap. OIL! Granted both liquids are in identical squirt bottles…but they are clearly labeled. Instead of drying, I have been generously greasing up the area to be treated, creating an oil slick. What a wing nut.

Bette is working at the table next to me. I lean over and whisper to her what I have just done.

She stops and looks me square in the face.

She says, "Jesus Christ. How many babies did you drop in your former career?"

The day before Thanksgiving, we learn "Buff and Bronze" which is a head-to-toe instant tanner. It is a self-tanning lotion that we smear all over each other to create the illusion of golden glowing tan skin. The morning we are doing this, there are several photographers present to get "action shots" for publicity photos for the school's PR campaign. It is crowded in the small upstairs body treatment room. The upstairs body treatment room has just been painted a soothing sage green color and has new wall-to-wall carpeting.

111

The picture on this page is a photo of Merrill that was taken at this very moment by these photographers for these pre-Holiday publicity shots. This photo is my favorite because I think Merrill looks very campy in this pose. This picture of Merrill was taken about ten minutes before my big "Buff and Bronze Disaster."

With the photographers jammed in the small room, it is very frenetic and confusing. The photographers are jockeying around the room vying for the most advantageous position and it is making me nervous. There are three tables stuffed in this room. That means six students and two instructors and three photographers. The Buff and Bronze lotion is a thick dark pudding of suspect ingredients, a veritable black soup of extracts of chamomile and goldenseal. Obviously, one can see where I am going with this.

Jett hands me a plastic cup full of the black pudding. I walk toward Merrill. I catch the toe of my cowboy boot on the leg of a facial table. I trip and pitch forward and the plastic cup flies out of my hand and hits the carpet. The rebound of the pudding sends it straight up in the air and it hits the wall at about six feet. The pudding starts dripping down the newly painted wall leaving a long dark fecal streak. I am horrified. The stuff is staining the wall in a very excretory manner. Shit.

Nobody misses a beat. Nobody even looks up. The photographers look nervously at each other, unsure of how to react.

All that the Beauty Girls say is, "Grace?"

"Yep, it's Grace."

"Nice going, Grace."

Jett rolls her eyes, sighs and heads off to get cleaning supplies.

The stains on the wall come clean. The new carpet does not. The brown trail is still evident. I notice it every day.

Some of the Beauty Girls decide that they want to bronze their breasts as well. It's a hard job but somebody's got to do it. There is quite a lot of bawdiness in the treatment room today. Lovely, perky breasts everywhere. I decline to bare my breasts myself because I don't want to scare these children with the reality of what happens to these erstwhile perky things once they pass the half-century mark.

Boobs heading South. Crossing the Mason Dixon Line. Mams eye to eye with one's navel. I will spare them the crushing visual.

When I am done bronzing Merrill, I think she is stunning. She looks like the Golden Goddess in Goldfinger. Absolutely a vision. How could she not be? Merrill could be sick with Mad Cow Disease and she'd still take your breath away.

I decide I do not like Buff & Bronze. We got off to a rough start, B&B and I. After Merrill coats me with it, I get a humongous herpes sore on my lower lip in response to the mysterious, toxic ingredients. I definitely will not be offering this service in my Women's Holistic Health Spa & Wine Bar.

~)(~

Thanksgiving is fun. There's a lot of yelling and screaming and swearing during a rousing game of Monopoly. After Thanksgiving, when I have a few days off, I find I can't stop cleaning my house. I strip all the beds, wash windows, put away summer clothes, do all the things I have been avoiding since I've been in school. I cook, clean, thaw, disinfect and launder. Compulsively. I have OCD with my house cleaning in my skimpy time off. As pathetic as it sounds, I am looking forward to going back to school so I can stop cleaning my house.

Believe it or not, I am looking forward to being back in the Convent.

Week Thirteen:

Queen of *WhoHa's*

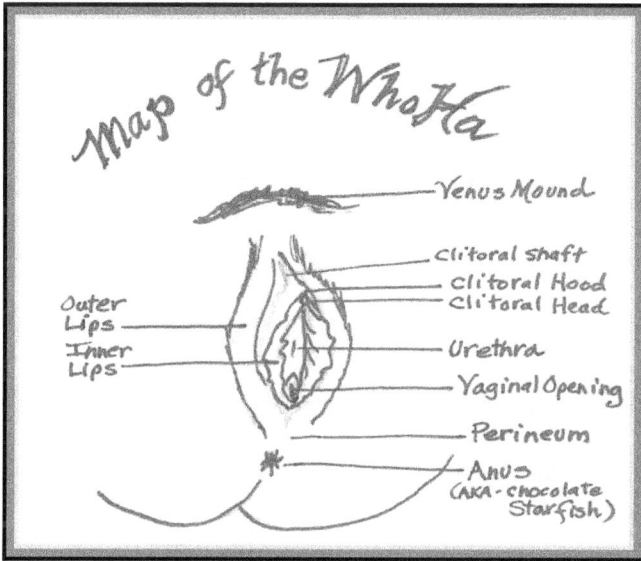

Map of the WhoHa

~)(~

Chapter 13

Nikita limps in from Thanksgiving vacation dragging her leg behind her. It is obvious she is in a lot of pain walking. She sits down gingerly and winces as she arranges her legs underneath her. She looks pale and shaky.

I think, "Now what?"

I say, "What's going on Mc Wienster?"

She rolls up her pant leg to expose a huge black and blue bruise running all the way up her leg. Then she shows me a matching bruise covering her entire left arm.

Nikita has crashed…again.

She says she was snowmobiling in Vermont with her posse this past weekend. They had been partying hard, as usual. It seems these accidents always have something to do with the conspicuous consumption of copious amounts of alcohol. Damn kids.

She is riding double with a girlfriend on the back of her sled. Her girlfriend is so sick and hung-over she is dead weight and is leaning heavily on Nikita's back. Nikita tries to negotiate a turn in the trail but her friend has passed out and Nikita misses the turn and flies down a ravine. She bombs down the hill, over a frozen stream and smashes straight into a large pine tree.

She has totaled her sled.

Up on the trail, the rest of her group sails by them, unaware of where they are.

Nikita is pretty banged up. Her friend is sprawled face down in the snow. The friend starts to come to, moaning about the pain.

Nikita has had it with her.

She yells, "Listen girlfriend, shut your piss flaps, you worthless piece of *dogshit*. Help me get us out of this smelly bunghole."

Nikita is lucky that only her sled is broken. It's a miracle that she's in one piece, probably too drunk to get really hurt. Due to the amount of liquid anesthesia, she's lucky she hasn't broken her lovely red neck.

I'm assuming this calls for more Suffering Bastards later on.

Midweek, a student from the class behind us—I guess we are considered Seniors now—shyly asks me if I will do her first Brazilian. As I have said, I am ambivalent about this current fashion of extreme *WhoHa* hair removal. The student says she wants to do this as a surprise birthday present for her boyfriend. I think this is bordering on pedophilia but I keep my opinion to myself.

The student also says she believes she should experience the pain first hand if she is going to offer this service to her clients.

I think, "OK. Fair enough. Let the de-fuzzing begin!"

The student gets undressed from the waist down and is lying on the body treatment table. I, on the other hand, have armored myself in a black plastic work apron because I know my penchant for getting sugar in my hair, my lab coat, my boots, somehow my bra.

The student is very soft-spoken and shy.

She says to me, "I chose you to do my Brazilian because I know you are so used to seeing *The Junk*."

I do not comprehend, "The Junk?"

She smiles sweetly, "Yeah. You know." She nods down below, "The Junk in My Trunk."

"Oh. Right." I finally get the reference to female genitalia. "That Junk."

Yeesh. Maybe I'm too old for this mid-life career change.

A Brazilian involves sugaring the entire "bikini" area, i.e., all hair is removed from the vulva, the mons pubis, the labia majora, the perineum and the anus. Every single hair. Pulled out systematically by the roots.

Yowcha!

Armed with my trusty spatula, I position myself between the student's legs and peer at her *WhoHa*. Her hair is modestly trimmed short, nice and neat. Perfect for a successful sugaring. I put on my new reading glasses, which by now have been bumped up to +2.00 so I can actually see what I'm doing.

Personally, I think this woman's "Junk" is absolutely adorable.

I sigh. I dip my spatula in the sugar pot and pull out some dripping hot sugar. It looks like honey. I lean over and smear a thin layer on the right side of her snatch, cover with the fabric strip, put pressure on to warm the sugar, then >>*Schwip!*>> all the pubic hair comes out.

The student lets out an astonished agonized gasp.

This is only the beginning.

The things we do for love.

Next comes the more delicate area along the labial folds. This is difficult to maneuver, as the labia tend to slide around unpredictably...sort of like trying to catch a slippery little salamander. I fold her nether lip down and hold it taut, trapping it before it can flee the sugar. I pull it tight so the lips won't stretch to the next county and I *Schwip!* before it can escape my grip. Clean as a baby's bottom...literally.

The student has hair around her anus that she wants to be gone. Some women don't want you messing with "that"—the Beauty Girls tactfully call it the "Chocolate Starfish"—but some want everything clean as a whistle. This is tricky to get in between the butt cheeks. I have the student hold her leg straight up in the air so I can maneuver. The student looks like a cat who is about to lick her own pussy.

As I bend over to move things around, I'm wondering, "Why do cats always pick the middle of the living room during a cocktail party to lick themselves with their leg sticking straight out?"

The next time you have a Brazilian, if you are wondering what your esthetician is thinking about when she's doing your service, there's a possibility that she is thinking about cats.

I have left the Venus Mound for last as that is the most sensitive area and can really be quite zippy. When I >>*Schwip!*>> the last of the student's hair off, I look up to see she has one big fat tear rolling down her cheek. Awww. She really has been a trooper. I hand her a mirror so she can see what she looks like.

Her mouth drops open and makes a perfect O in shock as she sees the baldness for the first time since puberty.

She says, "Oh my god. I look like a nine year old."

I say, "Yes you do."

I spray her nude *WhoHa* with Dermoplast and bid her good day.

A lot of the Beauty Girls say they like this because it makes them feel clean and silky and makes sex slipperier and more sensual. I think I know the real reason women decide to have a bald yoni. It's because it's a secret. You can be standing talking to someone in the grocery aisle and all of a sudden you remember that you are standing there with a pre-pubescent, shiny *WhoHa* and it makes you smile. It's such a trashy secret. It's wicked. It's a naughty secret pleasure hidden in a very private place.

Later that day I am sitting out back with Angel, Nikita and Bette. We are talking about this fad. Angel was in the Advanced Course ahead of us, so she has done tons of Brazilians. She is the Queen of *WhoHa's*. She says that one time a woman she was sugaring had an orgasm during the service.

I say, "Shut up! Are you sure?"

Angel says, "Absolutely. She was moaning and grimacing...and it wasn't from pain. It was from pleasure. She arched her back when she came."

Nikita says, "Hello? There is nothing sexy about getting your clit ripped off."

Bette chomps down on her knuckle in distress.

She says, "OK. That does it for me. I'm not doing them."

I shout, " 'I'm having what she's having!' I would have told her there's an additional $200 charge for that bonus service."

There is a lot of money in the complete hair removal business. I'm thinking of having cards made:

~ **BALD BEAVERS 'R US** ~

HAVE SPATULA. WILL TRAVEL.

FEES NEGOTIABLE

At the end of the week, we learn Moor Mud Body Wraps. The blurb on the Esthetics Institute's menu says, "This sterile mud's more than 1,000 plant extracts and trace elements are used to detoxify, as it draws out impurities and stimulates circulation. The world's most pure and potent source of healing mud leaves you feeling energized from head to toe."

The stuff comes from somewhere on the Austrian Moors. It is black and thick and smelly. All I can envision is wild foggy moors covered with ancient, prehistoric donkey dung that we are now smearing all over our bodies. It is messy and a total pain in the ass to remove. You need a jackhammer to get it off completely. Detoxify...*de-schmoxify*. I'd rather be toxic.

I have the Mud in a plastic container in the old turkey roaster that we use to keep all the wet towels warm. We need tons of towels to get the crap off. Soon the towels will be covered in gobs of the excremental black mud. Looks like a dog's breakfast.

I am setting up my body treatment table when I smell something burning. I turn to see a slight wisp of smoke coming from the old turkey roaster. *Godammit!* I throw the cover off and all the towels are scorched brown. The Moor Mud plastic container has melted into an unrecognizable shape, twisted and shrunken. The roaster's temperature control is set at the lowest setting…but the thing is so antiquated it has shorted out and is dangerously hot.

I am mad. I know that everyone is going to blame this on Grace…but in her defense, if the owners weren't so cheap, we'd have equipment that was made in this century.

Bette is in the room across the hall. She smells something burning. I tell her what has happened.

I say, "The owners are so cheap…if they don't invest in better equipment; they're going to burn the building down."

Bette says, "Right…they're such tight-asses, when they fart, only dogs can hear it."

I start to memorize the locations of the nearest fire extinguishers.

All the Beauty Girls are bare-naked ladies covered head to toe in the thick black mud. They are running to the showers in the upstairs dormitory with black faces and just the whites of their eyes and their laughing white teeth showing.

They look for all the world like Al Jolson singing "Mammy" in the Jazz Singer. I don't even bother to comment on this, as I know they're too young to have a clue as to what I am talking about. So I just stand there grinning as I watch them running around bare-assed in blackface.

I love these knuckleheads.

Week Fourteen:

Holy Mother of Pearl

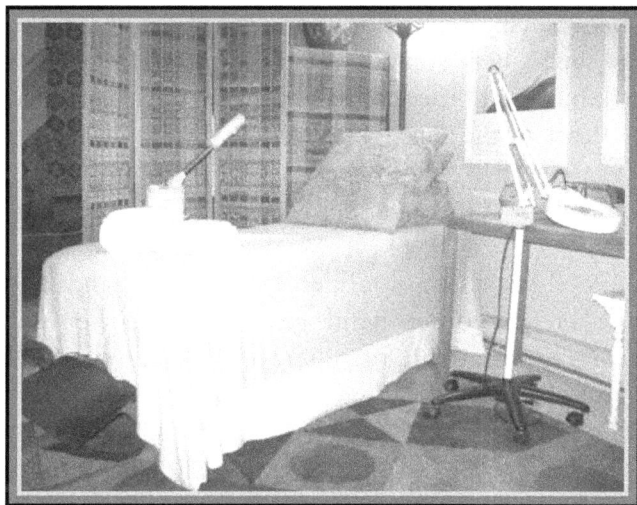

~ WRAPS and PAPS~
Natural Woman's Holistic Health Spa & Wine Bar

~)(~

Chapter 14

Rosacea.

Rosacea is all the industry "buzz" because it is the Skin Disorder du Jour. Apparently the incidence of rosacea is increasing at an alarming rate. Rosacea is chronic congestion primarily on the cheeks and nose, characterized by redness, dilation of blood vessels, and in severe cases, the formation of papules and pustules. The cause is unknown, but may be due to bacteria, mites, or fungus. Vasodilatation of the blood vessels [as with alcohol abuse] makes it worse. I think W.C. Fields had a flaming case of rosacea.

This week we are presenting our treatment plans for our hypothetical rosacea clients. I have interviewed my cousin, Berit, because she really does have rosacea and I'd like to be able to help her someday. Many interesting alternative, naturopathic and homeopathic approaches are discussed.

Pearl is the last of the Beauty Girls to present her rosacea case study.

I think, "Oh jesus, here we go"…but she proves me wrong.

Pearl stands up confidently with one hand in her lab coat pocket, the other hand gesturing with her pen. She knows exactly what she intends to do for her client. She has done her homework. Pearl's voice has changed; it is no longer squeaky and lispy. Even her face has matured significantly; the planes of her cheeks have become more angular. She has lost her baby fat.

Pearl's voice is clear and concise and strong as she outlines her treatment plan. No one else in the class has given the project this much thought. She presents several innovative, thoughtful ideas. Pearl stands tall and confident in her presentation and her knowledge. She is a young woman who has come into her power.

In fact, I am astounded. Pearl is kicking ass.

Mid-week, we have a freak snowstorm. By dawn there is at least a foot and a half of freezing snow. I keep calling the school to see if it is canceled, but it is not. The dog-and-pony show must go on, I guess. I slide down Dimond Hill in 4-wheel drive and see several cars off the road on my way to the Convent. The visibility is impossible. It is blowing and slippery and shitty.

Everything else in the city has been cancelled. I am concerned about the BGs who travel from a long distance. I can't believe the Mother Superior is making the kids come out in this weather. Pure stubborn orneriness.

The nearest free parking is a couple of blocks away from school. I am trudging in the blowing gusts with my head down bracing against the gale. I have on my fur-lined aviator hat with the flaps down but the snow still gets in my eyes. I am dragging my wheeled suitcase behind me in the slush but it catches every two feet and refuses to budge. I have to bump it up with my foot.

I am miserable.

Then I see something up ahead that makes me break into a huge grin.

Up ahead on the sidewalk in the snow is a lone set of wavering tracks from a wheeled suitcase. A little later on it is met by another set of thin wheelie lines coming from the right.

Then another set from the left. Finally another set from the right.

Four sets of wobbly tracks are going down the sidewalk, side-by-side in the snow.

I look down the block and I can barely see four Beauty Girls all in a row, leaning into the driving sleet, struggling to pull their suitcases behind them. They are hurrying in the storm, huddled together in a gaggle. Their slender coltish legs covered in black leggings are taking long strides in the slush in unison. And finally, like a flock of birds, they turn abruptly to the left and out of sight as they arrive at the entrance to the school.

I realize I have stopped in my tracks…what's this? I am crying. I am smiling and crying at the unexpected tenderness that this image has elicited. I realize it has been a very long time since I have cried from fondness. What a gift in the storm. All of a sudden the snow looks beautiful and magical to me.

Only five of us have made it to the Convent. I think the Mother Superior feels guilty about dragging us out in this weather because she turns the morning into her idea of a party. She has brought us Bread & Chocolate from the bakery across the street. This demonstration of appreciation is very out of character. Then she announces that she, *Herself*, is going to show us how to custom blend liquid foundation.

This is *some* party.

We are taught how to add tinted toner to the foundation to match base skin color; Mint to conceal redness, Lilac for sallowness, Sepia for darker skin types. After we measure and mix in beakers, we are ready for the application. The MS picks me for the demonstration, probably because of my Old Lady Skin. She believes she can give me that dewy, moist, "just kissed" look.

She dabs and schwipes and blots with a small sponge until she is satisfied. I swivel in my chair and look in the mirror. AAARRRRHHHH! The foundation is stuck in all the creases, accenting the wagon wheel ruts. Now I really do look like an old lady. I look like my late Aunt Gladys. Nope, worse. I look like Bette Davis in "Whatever Happened to Baby Jane?" This is terrifying. Shades of things to come.

At noon, Angel calls to say that she was trying to make it to school but went off the road on the ice. She is hysterical. The MS finally relents and school is closed for the rest of the day. We are released for the afternoon, so we all go to our local Mexican watering hole for Margaritas.

I love snowstorms.

On Friday afternoon, we are all jammed together in the Beauty Girls' far corner. There is tons of room in this hall, plenty of space to spread out, but for some reason we choose to sit all crowded together in the least amount of space possible. Probably so all our stuff gets intermingled and then we can bitch about it.

I have just done a Brazilian on a woman who has lost a ton of weight from gastric by-pass surgery, so the

130

conversation shifts to female genitalia and vaginas in particular.

Someone asks me the question, "So just how long is the vagina?" and I realize these guys have never even seen their internal workings, they've never checked themselves under the hood.

I say, "You guys, you mean to tell me you've never seen your cervix?"

"Nope."

"Gross."

Bette groans, "Here she goes again...Jesus. Enough with the cervix thing already, you know? Sick of this."

I grin. I salute her by lightly touching two fingers to my forehead, then I whip them down and out in front of me in the pelvic exam position. I say, "Carol Leonard...at your cervix!"

Mary covers her ears with her hands and buries her face in Milady.

I say, "But the cervix is so cute! It's this little round pink nubbin with a dimple in the middle, the cervical os. It's absolutely adorable. You guys have got to ask to see the next time you've got your feet in stirrups."

"Yah, with a cold metal thing shoved up your cooter." Nikita says delicately.

I say, "Wait a minute. Don't tell me you've never even felt your cervix?

"Nah uuuh."

"Oh my god, you guys." I can't believe this as the reality dawns on me. "Have you even put your fingers IN your vagina?"

"Get outta town."

"You're twisted, sistah."

Good Godfrey! I shake my head. "OK, here's the deal. Your assignment for tonight is to put your fingers in your *WhoHa* and feel your cervix. When you reach it, it feels like a nose, it's firm but moveable. And you can feel the little dimple in the middle of the 'nose'. It's awesome…and it's all yours!"

"But how do we know when we've found it…with all the other sthuff in there?" Pearl asks.

I am stunned silent for a second. Holy Mother of Pearl.

"What other 'stuff in there' Pearl? What the hell do you think you got in there? A carburetor? A radiator? A V-6? For *chrissake* Pearl!"

In the beginning of the week we had been so close…yet, now, so far.

I give up.

Thank gawd it's Friday.

Week Fifteen:

So Long Scrotum Eyes!

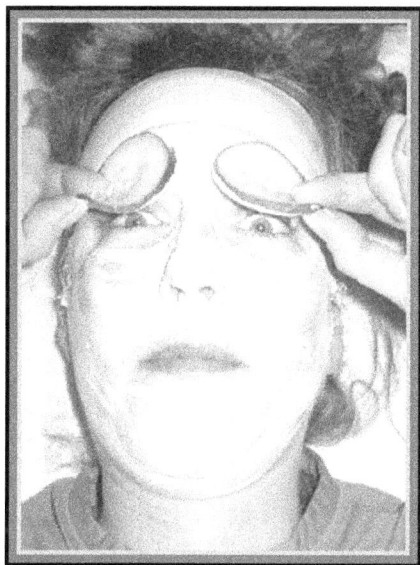

"Oh my god...they're gone!"

~)(~

Chapter 15

This week ushers in the advent of the Holiday Season. We are forced to decorate the Convent in festive holiday trappings. Lydia and I try to protest the quasi-religious implications, she because she is Jewish and I, because I am Unitarian, but it doesn't wash. We are indentured servants. We are forced to gaily wrap fake greenery and little lights and a bunch of other castaway glittery stuff around every available surface. The results look like a Bordello.

To celebrate the season, the Convent announces that we will be offering Champagne Facials and Harvest Grape Enzyme Pedicures to our clients.

Bah humbug.

I personally think it would be way more fun to actually drink the champagne instead of putting it on our faces, but I go with the flow. The Champagne Mask is intended to be a relaxing Finishing mask.

I have been assigned to be the first lucky recipient of the facial. Jacqueline is to be my Esthetician.

Jacqueline's baby bump is getting more pronounced with each passing day. It really is curvaceous, although I suspect a lot of times she exaggerates it and is sticking it out on purpose. She has just had an early ultrasound and brings the pix to school. She has also learned the gender of her baby. She is having a girl.

Jacqueline is very excited. She shows me the murky black and white images of her daughter.

"See? Isn't she cute?" Her eyes are dancing. "Look! It looks like she's waving to us!"

All I can see is a tiny image of a baby with an enormous rounded head. It looks like an Alien Baby curled up in there. A little miniature ET. A floating embryonic fish. Scary.

"Oh, how adorable!" I lie.

Jacqueline finishes the massage portion of my facial and is given the Champagne Facial mask powder in a pre-measured plastic cup from the locked instructor's cupboard. She mixes it with water and applies it to my face with a fan brush. She is instructed to leave it on for fifteen minutes.

It smells very strongly like sour grapes. We have the following conversation; I say, "Isn't sour grapes the same thing as Tartaric Acid?"

She says, "Yes, I believe so."

"Well, if it that's true, isn't Tartaric Acid considered an AHA? An acid peel? Don't those usually stay on for only a couple of minutes?"

She says, "The protocol card says 15 minutes. On a scale of one to five, how does it feel to you?"

I say, "One. It feels fine. No stinging. Just smells like a really rotten hobo wine. Mad Dog 20/20."

I listen to canned Christmas music. After fifteen minutes she starts to take it off.

She hesitates, "Um, Carol. You sure you don't feel anything? You're really pretty red under there."

Ouch. "Now that you mention it…Holy Crap!"

She sounds panicked. "Oh my god, Carol. Your face is all burned!"

"Owwwww. Owwwww. Owwwww." My new Mantra.

I am on fire.

Jett is called over. She takes one look, "Uh oh. Chemical burn."

She heads off for some ice. I never knew that someone that small could move that fast.

Jett comes back and packs my whole face in ice.

Searing pain. But the ice does start to diminish the heat. I feel a little nauseous.

My face looks like a red lobster. You can tell exactly where the mask was by the welts.

Jett applies a cooling cucumber gel mask and the pain begins to lessen.

She looks at the plastic container and sighs.

By accident, we have been given the Grape Pedicure Peel powder, the grape enzyme meant to dissolve calluses and corns on the feet. FEET! And even that was only supposed to stay on the feet for a few minutes.

My face is calming down somewhat. I still feel a little disoriented and sick. Mary offers to do a Healing Touch session for me to help me recover. She is wonderful. Her touch is focused and prayerful. I feel very blessed. I think Mary is a Mystic.

After this whole fiasco, I am too wiped out to face the crowd of students out back. I steal a pillow and a blanket from the body treatment room. I sneak upstairs and down the weird narrow dark hall to the empty back dorm bedroom. The beds are all stripped bare and the shades are drawn but it is quiet and dark in the room. I lie down with my pillow and blanket and curl up in a comfy ball. Yum.

I fall sound asleep.

Later in the day, Vivienne is in the downstairs bathroom penciling on her eyebrows getting ready to go bartend at The 99. She has tons of black mascara gobbed on her long dark lashes.

She says, "I am so exhausted I can barely function."

I say, "I just took a fabulous power nap in the upstairs back dorm room."

She stops penciling mid-arch. "Are you kidding me?"

I say, "Nope. Seriously, you should go take a nap."

She says, "What if we get caught?"

"We won't. There is yet another class behind us. They have their hands full. Besides, the instructors would never go down that hallway. It's too creepy."

She says, "Wow. This is awesome."

I say, "Yep. There's even a pillow and a blankie waiting for you."

"Done. I am so there. But don't tell anyone."

"I won't tell anyone. I promise. It will be our little secret."

She turns and levels me with her intense dark eyes, "Show me where he touched you on the doll."

The door closes behind her.

~)(~

At the end of the week, my face has healed completely. I wake up in the morning and look in the mirror and all the fine lines on my face have been burned off. Smooth as a baby's bottom.

And my Scrotum Eyes are half gone! The big edematous bags have been reduced to small fluid filled sacs. Now they're only about the size of Gummy Bears. I can't believe it. This is *the nuts*!

Tom comes into the bathroom yawning.

I say, "Tommy. Look! Look at my skin."

He peers closely at my face. "What?"

"Look how beautiful it looks!"

He pauses only a nanosecond, "Honey, you always look beautiful to me."

As I have said before, the boy is smooth.

Good save.

I am wondering how soon before I can do another Tartaric Acid Pedicure Peel on my face again.

Week Sixteen:

A Christmas Story

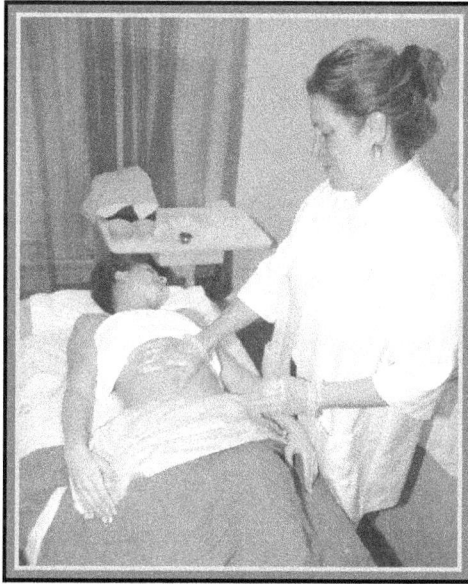

My classmates have begun to call me "Grace."

~)(~

Chapter 16

The end of this week is Christmas. The good news is that after this we have a whole week off. A whole week away from this place! It's amazing to me that even after all this time; I am still ambivalent about being here. The bad news is that the day we get back we have to take our mock State Board Written and Practical Exam for our grade. It appears our whole vacation will be spent preparing for this.

I am a little intimidated by the thought of the Practical Exam, only because I know I have the slim probability of being a total klutz. We are given pages of instructions as to how to prepare and pack and practice for this exam. Here's what we have to do flawlessly:

"Personal Prep & Appearance:"

1. Clean, professional clothing and lab coat
2. Hair off face; makeup done
3. No jewelry on hands; stud earrings (or none); no swinging necklace
4. No gum chewing
5. No perfume
6. No talking

Client Set-up & Protection—15 minutes
Cleansing the Face—10 minutes
Steaming the Face—10 minutes
Massaging the Face—10 minutes
Manual Extraction of the Forehead—10 minutes
Hair Removal of the Eyebrows [Tweezing, Soft Waxing]—15 minutes
Hair Removal of the Upper Lip [Hard Wax]—15 minutes
Facial Mask—10 minutes
Facial Makeup—20 minutes

I am going to use my kid sister, Wendy, as my model. I am going to have to practice this a bunch of times to get it down. Poor kid. I have always been able to talk my sister into anything. I've always experimented with new stuff on her. She says she's chronically in psychotherapy because of having me as her older sister.

It seems like this week everyone wants a pedicure done for the Holiday. I am beginning to loathe pedicures. Why does any woman bother? This is New Hampshire in winter for *godsake*. The best that can happen is that someone may see your toes for the split second that you take your foot out of your snowmobile boots before you jump into bed under the covers to get warm. I guess if it makes you feel sassy under the covers, then that's the point.

The women are having "Spa Pedicures" which the menu says is a special treatment for dry skin and "hard-working feet". It includes hot paraffin wax as a "Premium Product." The feet are dipped quickly three times in a vat of hot paraffin and then wrapped in plastic bags and then terry booties. The feet look like something from Madame Toussaud's.

I have finished the massage part of the pedi. I cross the room and unplug and lift up the big stainless steel paraffin heater that has six pounds of hot melted wax in it. As I come back across the room, I step on the long electric cord that is dangling from the heater and I trip forward. GODDAMMIT! I freeze in mid-motion. I'll be damned if I'm going to be the first one to spill a whole vat of wax on this new carpet. I grasp the heater tightly and as I am pitched forward I drop to my knees and twist my body and somehow roll over on my back and up the other side without spilling a drop.

The whole room is silently watching this.

Nikita yells, " 9.5 ! "

The room bursts into applause. I bow.

Grace 1. Heater 0.

~)(~

It is the last day of esthetics school before our Christmas vacation. We are going to have a whole week off from the Convent! I am so looking forward to getting out of this bloody place for an entire week that I can just about taste the Freedom.

The Pedicure room is packed with happy, noisy women. I am doing a pedi for a woman whose grown daughter is screeching in delight with the whole scene. They have all come en mass from the backwoods of Cow Hampshire somewhere...Newport, I think. They sound like they all just got off the skidder. The daughter's incessant screeching is giving me a headache. This is their first pedicure, Christmas gifts to each other I guess.

The daughter yells, "Maw! You still got chicken shit on your feet!"

I look down and she is absolutely right. The woman has gobs of poultry poop stuck in the crevices between her toes. This puts me in a very bad mood. I no longer loathe pedicures...I frigging HATE them.

In the late afternoon, just before the doors close, an elderly woman walks in for a pedicure. I am assigned to do it. Why do I always get the older women for this service? I am pretty upset. I hear the Beauty Girls out back chirping merrily as they pack up to go.

The old woman must be in her mid-eighties. She looks to be about my mother's age, if not older. She has gnarly yellow tubular nails with spongy mystery stuff underneath the nails. This is disgusting. Now I am getting really fed-up and pissed.

Out the front windows, I see the Beauty Girls leaving to go home for vacation. Pearl is power walking down the sidewalk with her rabbit-fur earmuffs and her wrap-around sunglasses on. She speed walks away from here like she is on an airport conveyer walkway. Away to Freedom. The other Beauty Girls are fleeing, trailing their wheeling suitcases behind them. They are all laughing. I see Vivienne doing her Three Stooges hopping backward down the sidewalk in the snow. Damn. This sucks big time.

I am so aggravated that I knick the woman's little toe by accident. She flinches but doesn't mention it. At first I see a tiny little pinhole of red but soon it grows and now she is bleeding profusely. I forgot to look to see if she was on blood thinners. Oh, crap. I try to stanch the red tide, but it keeps bleeding. I feel really bad for being so impatient.

The old woman is talking to me non-stop. I have already learned that her youngest son was killed in a motorcycle accident at age twenty-three. I also know her older son died of pancreatic cancer a month before her husband died two years ago.

It is the night before Christmas Eve. I am thinking about Tom, who is waiting for me to be done and call him so we can do last minute Christmas shopping and go out for dinner.

I finish the nail polish and the woman announces that it is not dry enough for her to leave, so she sits and continues to talk. She says she grew up in Manchester…blah, blah. We sit there as the polish dries. I can hear a clock ticking. I am alone in this place with this old woman and it is the night before Christmas Eve.

It starts to get dark outside. There are tiny twinkling white lights on the mantle. Christmas music comes on the CD player, and my anger softens. Suddenly it dawns on me. Duh. This woman is lonely. She has no one who loves her who is waiting for her to come home so they can have a drink and go out Christmas shopping together. I look at her. She is here with me on the night before Christmas Eve and I have just painted her toes a sassy red Holiday color.

I take a long deep inhalation.

I say, "Tell me, Doris, what was Manchester like when you were a young girl?"

~)(~

~ Merry Christmas to Us All ~

Week Seventeen:

The Last Week

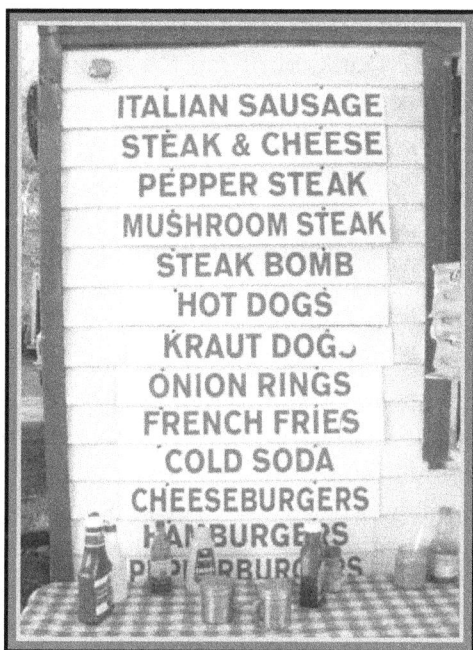

ITALIAN SAUSAGE
STEAK & CHEESE
PEPPER STEAK
MUSHROOM STEAK
STEAK BOMB
HOT DOGS
KRAUT DOG
ONION RINGS
FRENCH FRIES
COLD SODA
CHEESEBURGERS
HAMBURGERS
PEPPERBURGERS

The Weirs Beach Diet

~)(~

Chapter 17

This is the last week and soon I'll be out of this god-forsaken hole for good. I can't believe I made it. It seems like an eternity, and yet, it seems like only yesterday that I was scared shitless of Vivienne. Vivienne! I thought I'd be ecstatic to be done…but this feels strangely anticlimactic.

The rest of the Beauty Girls are continuing on for the Advanced Program. It's an additional three months. Three months of being instructed by the Mother Superior herself.

Nine months total...like a pregnancy. No thanks. I just want to get my license and begin working.

But now I feel kind of sad about finishing. I'm going to really, really miss these guys.

However, even this week, we are still bored out of our girdles. Half of the time we are waiting for "real clients" to do services for, so we are out back biding our time with our thumbs up our noses, eating chocolate. Jacqueline entertains us by baring her belly, and we all sit around mesmerized, staring and waiting for her daughter to move. From across the room, I see her girl stick her foot out dramatically. We all clap and cheer as Jacqueline's stomach does another huge rock and roll. Jacqueline is obsessively tactile with her "baby bump." She can't keep her hands off her in-utero daughter, touching, patting, massaging her. I think this is going to be a much-loved baby.

By Wednesday afternoon the Beauty Girls are huddled in our regular spot in the far southwest corner of the gymnasium—as far away from the Head Table as possible. Farthest away from the Mother Superior and the instructors so they can't hear us trash-talking them. It's slow out front and we are wicked bored, as usual when it's dead.

The instructors are all on the South Beach Diet and they are being Bitches from Hell. I'm trying to get all the students to sign a petition to demand that the instructors eat some frickin' carbs before we have to put them out of their misery. We're scheming about ways to get them to eat some French fries, bread, pasta, anything with glucose—so they will stop being so damn mean.

Nikita says, "What those *be-atches* need is a visit from the Red Tide. I say we fuck shit up! *Hell* yeah!"

She pumps her fist in the air over her head and yells, "ATTICA! ATTICA!"

152

I say, "Yeah right. Maybe if we bring in some beer and pork rinds, they'll turn their South Beach Diet into the Weirs Beach Diet."

At the end of the week we have our "mock state board" to prepare us for the real thing. After the exam is over I am sitting at our table in Beauty Girl corner when I look up to see a very handsome young man shyly standing in the lobby holding a dozen long-stemmed red roses. I nod toward him and the Beauty Girls turn around and gawk. Pearl jumps up and runs toward the boy and throws her arms around him. I'm guessing this is her live-in boyfriend, Jake. I find it interesting to see what the girls' partners look like. I'm intrigued.

Jake looks a little embarrassed.

All the Beauty Girls say, "Awww."

He leans over and kisses her, hands her the roses, whispers something to her and ducks out the door.

Pearl is beaming. She comes back with the roses, sits down in the middle of us and opens up his card.

She reads, "Dear Baby Girl, Congrats on passing your test! I'm so proud of you." Pearl stops. Her voice is husky with emotion.

Bette is sitting next to her and she is blubbering.

"Oh my god," Bette flips up her glasses and dabs her eyes, "This is just the cutest damn thing."

On Friday afternoon, the very last day, the MS holds us hostage and will not release us until exactly 4:31 PM. This is such a moronic practice. The Beauty Girls are pissed. They want out of here.

"This is total bullshit." Lydia growls.

As we are being herded down the hall and out the door to sign out, someone starts to Moo.

"Moooooo. Moooooo."

Someone else makes a sound like a sheep.

"Baaaaaaaa. Baaaaaaa."

Nikita whinnies.

We keep shuffling slowly out the door like cattle out the chute.

"Mooooooo. Mooooooo."

"Baaaaaaaaa. Baaaaaaaaa."

I make a sound like a duck.

"Quaaack. Quaaaack. Quaaaack."

They all stop and look at me…but no one has the energy to comment.

It's official. We've all lost our freaking minds in this place. But…we're done and "We're OFF! *like a prom dress*" as the Beauty Girls like to say.

~)(~

All the Beauty Girls passed the State Board Examination. Pearl got the highest grade of all. All passed, that is, except Shrimpy. Shrimpy disappeared in the last month of school and no one knows where she went.

My sincere thanks, deep gratitude and love go to all the Beauty Girls—thank you for being who you are. I have to honestly say, if you hadn't been so unbelievably funny and sassy and irreverent and kind, I never would have made it past the first week. I stayed because you made the experience tolerable and every other thing out of your mouths made me laugh deep down in my soul. You are true Goddesses of Beauty. May you all find your hearts desire.

Epilogue:

Wraps & Paps

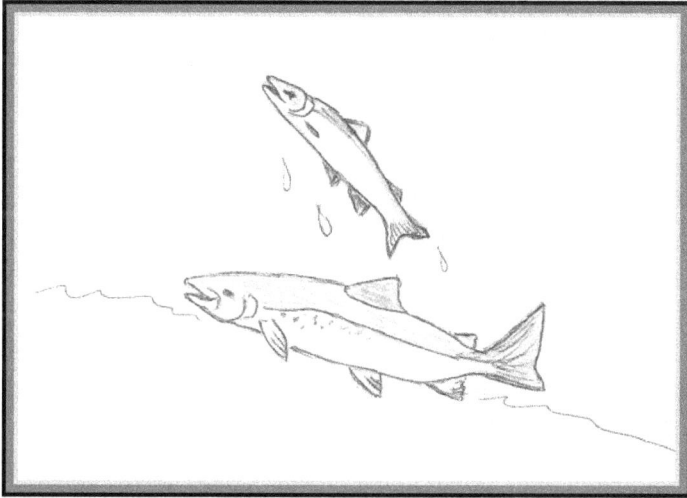

The Uncontrollable Urge to Swim Upstream.

~)(~

Epilogue

I have done it! I am now officially licensed as an Esthetician and as a NH Certified Midwife and I have opened my adorable little shop in Hopkinton. It's called:

~ WRAPS and PAPS ~
Natural Woman's Holistic Health Spa
& Wine Bar

I decide to have a "Grand Opening" to celebrate my perseverance. I am offering a FREE PAP SMEAR with the first ten facials. I have struck a good arrangement with my receiving lab to read the Paps and I place an ad in our local paper announcing the party.

On the day of the party, the first woman to arrive is a very elegant and refined woman in her late 70's, Mrs. Rutherford. Mrs. Rutherford hops right up on to my exam/facial table for her exam. She is such a good sport. She is ensconced in large brocade pillows as I check her blood pressure and ask about yearly mammograms. I gently do her pelvic exam and her Pap, and we have a discussion about her health in general.

When I have completed her exam, I take festive lavender and sage colored ribbons and tie a bow around the handle of the clean plastic speculum and give it to Mrs. Rutherford as a party favor. This absolutely cracks her up, she says this is the most unique party favor she has ever received in her life and can't wait to show her husband.

Now Mrs. Rutherford turns around lying with her head toward me and we begin the facial. The mask I am using is French and the container says it is a phenomenal anti-aging mask with ingredients of natural green clay, extract of avocado oil, borage oil, marine collagen, Vitamin E and Integral DNA.

As I always do, I have tested this mask on myself and I absolutely love it.

As part of my treatment, I tell her the ingredients that are in the mask as I am using it. Thus we get to the "Integral DNA" part.

She asks, "Whose DNA?"

I hesitate for a nanosecond, then I say, "Oh, I'm sure it's derived from a plant source."

But I have a nagging sense of doubt. I almost always thoroughly research the ingredients in the products I use. How could I have just "skipped" the DNA part?

On Friday the new Universal catalogue comes in the mail. I am flipping through the skincare part, shopping, when I get to the new mask. There it says, "Integral refers to the fact that the DNA polymer remains unbroken through the careful process of extraction. This ensures it maintains its regenerative properties, holding 10,000 times its volume in water, working to minimize wrinkles, dryness, roughness, fragility, and other visible signs of aging. Integral DNA is a highly evolved, pharmaceutical-grade biological extract derived from salmon milt."

"What the heck is salmon milt?" I ask Tom.

Tom says, "I have a bad feeling about this."

We look up "milt" in the dictionary. The dictionary says, "the male reproductive glands of fishes when filled with secretion; also: the secretion itself."

Oh Dear God, please, please, *please*, tell me I haven't just smeared Mrs. Rutherford's face with *fish spooge*.

I Google the words "salmon milt".

Yep, there it is, my mask is the fourth item down. "Atzen's Biologique: Salmon Milt-based Skin Care. The secret ingredient? A biopolymer extracted from salmon milt [sperm]. Called Integral DNA™, Atzen says this extract is credited with the ability to regenerate severely damaged skin tissue, even that from a burn. Integral refers to the fact that the DNA polymer remains intact – not broken or damaged – during extraction, allowing the Integral DNA to hold 10,000 times its volume in water."

Alrighty then. The Ethical Esthetician in me has a long debate about the responsibility here. Do I tell her? Do I not tell her? I decide to call her.

"Hello, Mrs. Rutherford?" I say over the phone. "Remember the other day when you asked me about the DNA in that mask? Well, it turns out that the source is from salmon milt, which is…um, what I'm trying to say is, it was from salmon sperm."

There is dead silence for a couple of beats. I am holding my breath. What if she is really upset by this?

Then …Mrs. Rutherford speaks.

"Well," she says, "I have been telling my friends that ever since I had that facial with you, I've had the uncontrollable urge to swim upstream."

Life is good. Life is very, very good.

Beauty Girls Definitions

Beef Curtains. The frontal wedgie. The zipper muffin. Garments with a tight central seam that serve to divide the labia majora into a visibly protruding cleft bulge.

Bubblegum. A man's "package." The external genitalia of the male (and the Creator of All Things has some serious explaining to do.)

Bunghole. See Chocolate Starfish.

Camel Toes. The lips of the labia majora, as seen through too tight running pants, resembling the large hooves of even-toed ungulates or camels. (Conversely, male organs shown through too tight clothes are called Moose Knuckles.)

Cervical os. The opening of the cervix into the vagina [external os].

Cervix. In gynecology, pertaining to the cervix uteri or neck of the uterus; it is about 1 inch long and opens into the vagina.

Chocolate Starfish. The anus and immediate surrounding area.

Clitoris. In women, a small sensitive organ consisting of erectile tissue, situated at the junction of the labia minora. It is a complex and wonderful organ that is designed for one specific purpose—pleasure.

Cooter. Slang for the vagina.

Dropping the kids off at the pool. Bowel movement.

The Junk. The external genitalia or external organs of reproduction (can be either male or female.)

Piss flaps. The canal through which urine is discharged from the bladder.

The Red Tide. Menstrual period.

Speculum. A metal or plastic instrument used to open up the vagina to view the hidden, adorable cervix. (A speculum looks like a duck-bill.)

Spooge. The male secretion of seminal fluid from the prostate gland (also found in fish.)

Uterus. The womb: a powerful, pear-shaped, orbed, muscular organ situated in the pelvic cavity between the bladder and the rectum. It is by far the most amazing organ of any creation of the Universe.

Venus Mound. (*mons veneris*) The mounded area covered with hair over the pubes in a woman.

WhoHa. The Beauty Girls favorite word for the beautiful female genitalia.

ACKNOWLEDGEMENTS

I would like to thank Christine Pinheiro Silva for absolutely, ruthlessly, goading this project on. Without her, The Beauty Girls would never have seen the light of day. Her book, *The Step-By-Step Guide to Self-Publishing for Profit!* (PassKey Publications, 2009) was my bible in navigating Amazon's CreateSpace program for self-publishing. Her belief in my writing, and the novel idea that I could actually be successful at it, was my inspiration to let it fly.

Also, my colleague and editor, Jane Hunter Munson. Thank you for reining me in when things got too "over-the-top." I apologize profusely for using so many Capitalized Words. I don't know What Got In To Me.

Lastly, my BFF, Kudra MacCaillech. You've always teased me about, "Careful or you'll end up in my novel." Now you're on my cover. Ha! That's hilarious, girlfriend.

About Carol Leonard

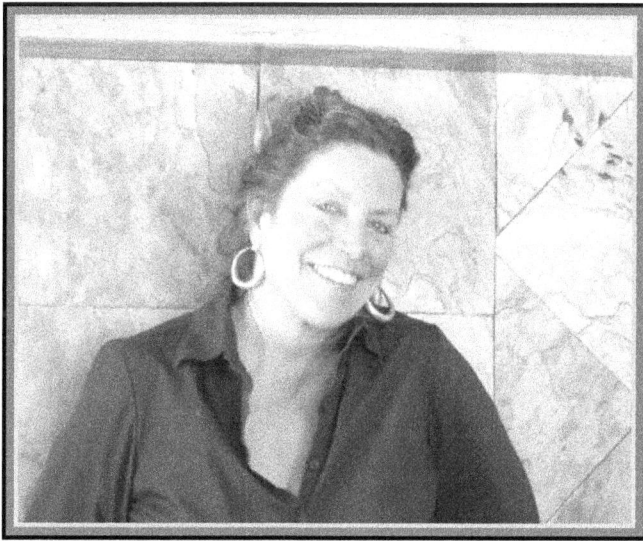

AUTHOR NOTE

Carol Leonard and her husband, Tom Lajoie, have a 400 acre parcel of land in Ellsworth, Maine, that they are making into a tree farm. They are doing sustainable harvesting and Tom has a saw mill there. They have named the land Bad Beaver Farm. For further information and for speaking engagements, go to: *www.BadBeaverFarm.com*.

To order additional SIGNED copies of *The Beauty Girls*, please go to: *www.beautygirlsbook.com*.

www.ingramcontent.com/pod-product-compliance
Lightning Source LLC
Chambersburg PA
CBHW061723020426
42331CB00006B/1072